2

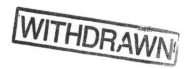

KT-162-224

WITHDRAWN

Caring for Children
Towards Partnership with Families

USING NURSING MODELS SERIES

General Editors:
Jane E. Schober MN, SRN, RCNT, DipN Ed, DipN(Lond), RNT.
Principal Lecturer in Nursing, Department of Health and Community Studies, School of Health and Life Sciences, Leicester Polytechnic.

Christine Webb BA, MSc, PhD, SRN, RSCN, RNT.
Professor of Nursing, Department of Nursing, University of Manchester.

The views expressed in this book are those of the authors of individual chapters and do not necessarily reflect the opinions of the series editors.

Caring for Children
Towards Partnership with Families

Edited by

Alison While
BSc, MSc, PhD, RGN, RHV.

Senior Lecturer
Department of Nursing Studies
King's College
University of London.

Edward Arnold
A division of Hodder & Stoughton
LONDON MELBOURNE AUCKLAND

© 1991 Alison While

First published in Great Britain 1991

British Library Cataloguing in Publication Data

While, Alison
Caring for children and their families.
1. Children. Nursing
I. Title   II. Series
610.7362

ISBN 0–340–51840–5

Whilst the advice and information in this book is believed to be true
and accurate at the date of going to press, neither the author nor the
publisher can accept any legal responsibility or liability for any errors
or omissions that may be made.

In particular (but without limiting the generality of the preceding
disclaimer) every effort has been made to check drug dosages;
however, it is still possible that errors have been missed. Furthermore,
dosage schedules are being continually revised and new side-effects
recognized. For these reasons the reader is strongly urged to consult
the drug companies' printed instructions before administering any of
the drugs recommended in this book.
   All names of patients have been changed to protect their identity.

Typeset in 10/12 Ehrhardt by TecSet Ltd, Surrey.
Printed and bound in Great Britain for Edward Arnold, a division of
Hodder and Stoughton Limited, Mill Road, Dunton Green,
Sevenoaks, Kent TN13 2YA by The Bath Press, Avon

Contents

Contributors

Gillian Chapman BSc, MSc, PhD, RGN, RSCN. Nursing Officer, Department of Health, London

Shirley Dean BA, MSc, RGN, RM, RHV, RHVT. Senior Lecturer, Department of Health and Paramedical Studies, West London Institute of Higher Education.

Yvonne Diment BA, MSc, RGN, RM, RHV. Community Health Service Manager, North Hertfordshire.

Barbara Elliott BNurs, RGN, RSCN, RHV, DN Cert. Clinical Nurse Specialist (Research), Booth Hall Children's Hospital, Manchester.

Kathryn Jones BSc, RGN, RSCN. Nurse Teacher, Charles West School of Nursing, Hospital for Sick Children, Great Ormond Street, London.

Sally Kendall BSc, RGN, RHV. Senior Lecturer, Department of Nursing, Buckinghamshire College of Higher Education.

Hazel MacKenzie BSc, RGN, RSCN, DN Cert. Ward Sister, Royal Hospital for Sick Children, Edinburgh.

Susan Ritter MA, RGN, RMN. Lecturer in Psychiatric Nursing and Honorary Clinical Nurse Specialist, Institute of Psychiatry, University of London.

Alison While BSc, MSc, PhD, RGN, RHV. Senior Lecturer, Department of Nursing Studies, King's College, University of London.

Mark Whiting BNurs, MSc, RGN, RSCN, DN Cert., RHV. Senior Nurse Manager (Paediatric and Neonatal Care), Waltham Forest Health Authority.

Dorothy Whyte BA, PhD, RGN, RSCN, RM, RNT, RHV. Lecturer, Department of Nursing Studies, University of Edinburgh.

Preface

This book is designed to complement the other books already published in the 'Using Nursing Models' series. The chapters are oriented exclusively around the care of children and their families, and attempt to demonstrate the potential of the application of theoretical models to the provision of health care delivery.

Demographic data is conclusive in demonstrating an increase in older people in the population relative to other age groups. This has clear implications for health and social care provision. However, it has to be remembered that children of today are the productive workforce and carers of tomorrow, and therefore it is imperative that continued efforts are made to improve the quality of care given to children.

The chapters draw upon a variety of theoretical models, some of which may not be regarded as strictly nursing models. However, the contributors have sought to use models which they consider most appropriate to their care situation and would argue that their case study approaches demonstrate the suitability of their model choice. Indeed, they may introduce alternative models to the readers of this book and inspire improved care as a consequence.

Each contributor is an experienced health care professional and attempts to develop a limited critical review of material drawing upon relevant research and professional expertise. It is hoped that the breadth of the chapters provides both interest and inspiration – if we assist health care professionals in their striving towards becoming reflective practitioners, we will have succeeded in our aim.

Alison While
London, 1990.

Note: *Due to the need for confidentiality, fictitious names have been used in the case studies and there is no intention to imply similarity with any known child or their family.*

Acknowledgements

I should like to thank all the contributors for their chapters without whom this book would never have emerged. I am also grateful to the support of editorial staff at Edward Arnold. The helpful comments of the series editors were also much appreciated.

Finally, I should like to thank all those with whom I live and work for their tolerance –

Frances, our trusty nanny;
William and Edward, two 'helpful' boys;
Philip, an inspiring life companion;
Colleagues in the Department of Nursing Studies, King's College and especially Yvonne Dennis, for managing to survive poor handwriting, telephone calls and an office move.

1

Introduction
Alison While

In earlier times, childhood was thought of as an incomplete and inadequate form of the adult state (Aries, 1973). However, childhood is now recognized as a period of human experience in its own right, and indeed, there is a general acknowledgement that childhood experience is an important factor in the development of the later adult.

The issue of the detrimental effects of hospitalization upon children, especially young children, was first raised in 1946 (Curtis Report, Ministry of Health). The Platt Report (Ministry of Health, 1959) supported the conclusions of the Curtis Report and advocated that the mother and child should not be separated if this could be avoided. The Platt Report further recommended that children should be treated at home whenever possible and noted that:

> 'Too few local authorities as yet provide special nursing schemes for home care of children and the extension of such schemes should be encouraged.'
>
> (para. 18.)

Later, the Court Report (DHSS, 1976) placed a much greater emphasis upon home care than previous government documents:

> 'The importance of the family must be reflected in the organization and delivery of health care services for children.'
>
> (para. 5.5)

A desire to improve family health care support in the community has been restated on several occasions (Ministry of Health, 1971; DHSS, 1981; Department of Health, 1989).

This emphasis upon the potential contribution of home care is founded upon the wealth of research that indicates that hospitalization of young children has far-reaching psychological effects (Spence, 1947; Bowlby, 1953; Robertson, 1958; Brain and Maclay, 1968; Rutter, 1972; Butler and Golding, 1986). It has also been demonstrated that children experience less emotional trauma if their mothers remain with them during hospitalization (MacCarthy *et al.*, 1962; Hally *et al.*, 1977; Belson, 1981; Sainsbury *et al.*, 1986). Child health care provision is therefore concerned to provide child-centred family care designed to reinforce the ability of parents, so that the child may receive the best possible care in the circumstances.

In acknowledgement of the current philosophy underpinning child health provision, this book attempts to provide exemplars of practice based upon different theoretical models. Pearson and Vaughan (1986) have suggested that model-based practice is an important element in effecting change in the quality of care provision, and indeed, McFarlane (1986) has argued that:

> '. . . practice which is shorn of any theoretical basis and which does not allow its theoretical foundations to grow is not a practice discipline. It

is a ritualized performance unrelated to health care needs of individuals and society.'

(p.1)

However, there are now an increasing number of models available for the practitioner and although some of these models share certain aspects, their conceptualization of the nature of people may vary considerably. This poses the problem of model selection. For the erudite practitioner who wishes to commence a detailed epistemological analysis of the underpinnings of four of the most famous American model architects (King, Orem, Rogers and Roy), I recommend *The Nature of Theoretical Thinking in Nursing* (Kim, 1983). However, few practitioners have either the inclination or the time to devote many hours to the development of this level of understanding and, therefore, a few words about model selection may prove helpful to the reader.

Firstly, a model is limited by the values and beliefs of its proposer and in view of this, it is most unlikely that any one model will be appropriate for all care situations. Chalmers (1989) has set out the following criteria for the evaluation of models: clarity; consistency; simplicity/complexity; scope; utility and social congruence, and when applied, these criteria should help identify an appropriate model for use in practice. Webb (1986) has argued that:

'Practising nurses themselves . . . must evaluate nursing models and their usefulness in patient care.'

(p.1)

Occasionally, an inappropriate model may be selected, and if this adversely affects the potential of care it will be regrettable if the selection of a model for practice is not reversible!

The common division between community and institutional care has been deliberately underplayed in this book, with both types of care well represented among the chapters. Another common problem of health care provision for children is the supremacy of physical care over psychological care, with the effect that many registered sick children's nurses have a very limited knowledge of child mental health problems and their care. It is hoped the inclusion of two chapters which specifically examine the special needs of these children will help to redress the balance.

Jolly (1981) has asserted that:

'The challenge of paediatric nursing today is in meeting the needs of the whole child. This means not only attending to his physical care, but also paying attention to his thoughts, his feelings, and his need for his family.'

(p.3)

The chapters in this book attempt to demonstrate how this challenge may be successfully met, and it is hoped that practitioners will be able to draw upon the theoretical models described in order to enhance their practice. It is not expected that practitioners will necessarily agree with what the contributors have written; however, if this book encourages thinking and debate then it has succeeded in its purpose.

References

Aries P (1973). *Centuries of Childhood*. Penguin, Harmondsworth, Middlesex.
Belson P (1981). Alternatives to hospital care. *Nursing*; 23: 1015–16.
Bowlby J (1953). *Child Care and the Growth of Love*. Pelican, Harmondsworth, Middlesex.
Brain DJ and Maclay I (1968). Controlled study of mothers and children in hospital. *British Medical Journal*; 1: 278–80.
Butler NR and Golding J (eds) (1986). *From Birth to Five*. Pergamon, Oxford.
Chalmers HA (1989). Theories and models of nursing and the nursing process. *Recent Advances in Nursing*; 24: 32–46.
Department of Health (1989). *Caring for People*. HMSO, London.
DHSS (1976). *Fit for the Future*. The Report of the Committee on Child Health Services. Cmnd 6684. Chairman: Professor SDM Court. HMSO, London.
DHSS (1981). *Care in the Community*. HMSO, London
Hally MR, Holohan A, Jackson RH, *et al.*(1977). Paediatric home nursing scheme in Gateshead. *British Medical Journal*; 1: 762–64.
Jolly J (1981). *The Other Side of Paediatrics*. Macmillan, London.
Kim HS (1983). *The Nature of Theoretical Thinking in Nursing*. Appleton-Century-Crofts, New York.
MacCarthy D, Lindsay M and Morris I (1962). Children in hospital with mothers. *Lancet*; 24 March: 603–8.
McFarlane J (1986). The value of models for care, in Kershaw B and Salvage J (eds), *Models for Nursing*. John Wiley, Chichester.

Ministry of Health (1946). *Report of the Care of Children Committee.* (Curtis Report). HMSO, London.

Ministry of Health (1959). *The Welfare of Children in Hospital.* Report of Central Health Services Council. Chairman: Sir Harry Platt. HMSO, London.

Ministry of Health (1971). *Hospital Facilities for Children.* Memo No. 22. HMSO, London.

Pearson A and Vaughan B (1986). *Nursing Models for Practice.* Heinemann, London.

Robertson J (1958). *Young Children in Hospital.* Tavistock, London.

Rutter M (1972). *Maternal Deprivation Reassessed.* Penguin, Harmondsworth, Middlesex.

Sainsbury CPQ, Gray OP, Cleary J *et al.,* (1986). Care by parents of their children in hospital. *Archives of Disease in Childhood*; **61**: 612–5.

Spence JC (1947). Care of children in hospital. *British Medical Journal*; 1: 125–30.

Webb C (ed) (1986). *Women's Health.* Hodder and Stoughton, London.

2

A home visit by the health visitor using Bandura's theory of self-efficacy
Sally Kendall

Introduction

The concern of health visiting has always been the improvement and promotion of child health. From its inception as a voluntary service in the 19th century public health movement to its present day universal role with families, the profession has consistently aimed at reducing infant mortality and morbidity and promoting the welfare of children within the family context through health education, health advice and counselling. The main structures which the health visitor currently has available to her to try to meet this aim are the child health clinics and the home visit. This chapter will concentrate on the home visit as a structure for assessing the needs and planning the care for one family.

It is important to emphasize that whilst the health visitor is concerned with the health of a child, this can only be assessed within the psychosocial and biological context of the family. For example, the dependency relationship between an infant and her mother will dictate, to some extent, the child's health status in relation to the mother's. Thus, failure to thrive in a young baby may be due to the fact that the mother is depressed and fatigued and unable to produce sufficient breast-milk. Of course, there may be other medical explanations, but the role of the health visitor is to observe and assess what is happening in the whole family, not just to survey the child in isolation. For this reason, health visitors have been referred to as 'family visitors' (Clark, 1973).

Current thinking in health visiting appears to fall into two areas. There is one school of thought which suggests that health visiting has concentrated for long enough on the needs of the child: present day infant mortality rates do not warrant a universal service, and a targeted service based on the health needs of the whole community should be considered (Goodwin, 1988). There is another school of thought which proposes that the needs of children in the community remain a priority which health visitors have the expertise to address. This view has been put forward by researchers such as Barker (1984), who acknowledges the need for continued child surveillance programmes, and Bedford (1988), who advocates the need to increase immunization uptake. Whatever future direction the profession takes, there is agreement that the assessment of child health will continue to be a part of the health visitor's role in one form or another.

The context of the care plan

The case under consideration in this chapter is based on a real family situation, although the assessment and care plan are hypothetical since the author was not in a position to implement the proposed theoretical framework (Bandura's theory of self-efficacy 1977b) at the time. During a research study on client participation in health visiting

(Kendall, in progress) the author collected a large amount of data on the approach used by health visitors to assess family health needs and on the perceptions of the clients of a home visit. The overall findings indicated the health visitors rarely assess client's needs from the client's perspective but follow an agenda usually dictated by a child development model, and that as a consequence of this, parents had vague perceptions about the home visit which frequently did not match with the health visitor's. This led the author to consider possible theoretical frameworks which would enable the health visitor to assess from the client's perspective, thereby leading to more effective care. The family described below serve to illustrate that process.

Dawn and Trevor Harris lived in a two bed-roomed maisonette in an outer suburb of north London. Trevor worked in a small local industry which manufactured electrical goods. Dawn gave up her job as a VDU operator after their first son, Michael, was born. Michael was three years old at the time of the visit and the second baby, Jamie, was four months old. The family had lived in the area since Dawn and Trevor were married four years previously, having moved away from Dawn's family in London. Trevor's family lived in Kent. Trevor worked long hours to get as much overtime as he could as the couple wanted to buy their own home. This usually included week-end work. Dawn, therefore, saw little of him during the day and he arrived home late, often tired and irritable. Whilst recognizing the need for Trevor's long working week, Dawn was finding it quite difficult managing two children with very little support from either her husband or family. Michael was a particular problem to her because his behaviour had altered noticeably since the arrival of Jamie. He woke frequently at night, had reverted to wetting the bed and had on occasions behaved violently towards the baby. Whilst the general family history was known to the health visitor, she was not aware of the development of this problem prior to her visit. Her objectives for visiting the family were primarily to discuss immunization for Jamie, which had not started, and weaning him onto solid food. This family has been selected to illustrate the application of Bandura's (1977b) theory of self-efficacy because it became clear that the main health needs

of the children were being directly influenced by Dawn's capacity to cope with the situation.

Bandura's theory of self-efficacy

Before looking in detail at the assessment of this family, it is necessary to explore the major constructs of Bandura's theory, their relevance to health visiting and thus the rationale for adopting this framework.

Self-efficacy theory is derived from Bandura's (1977a) work in social learning theory. Social learning theory suggests that cognitive processes play a prominent role in the acquisition and retention of new behaviour. Motivation is seen in terms of capacity to cognitively represent the future consequences of behaviour, and thus behaviour is affected largely by the creation of expectations that the action will produce anticipated benefits or avert future difficulties.

Self-efficacy theory as proposed by Bandura (1977b), is a conceptual framework for analysing and explaining changes in behaviour. The theory postulates that people's perceptions of their capabilities affect how they behave, their level of motivation, thought patterns and emotional reactions to taxing situations. Self-efficacy theory describes one common mechanism through which people exercise influence over their own motivation and behaviour. Bandura suggests that people tend to avoid situations or activities which they believe exceed their capabilities and they attempt behaviour which they feel capable and confident of performing. Personal judgement of self-efficacy also determines the effort one will expend in the face of obstacles and how one will respond emotionally. The belief that one can influence events tends to reduce uncertainty and anxiety. On the other hand, dependency can set in when one feels incapable of influencing personally significant events. People respond to anxiety-inducing events in a number of ways. They can seek information in an effort to reduce uncertainty, acquire the skills necessary for achieving control, or try to avoid the situation altogether. In some situations, for example serious illness, the exercise of personal control carries heavy responsibility and risk. In such a situation, Bandura suggests that the individual may be willing to relinquish personal control in order to 'free themselves of the performances and hazards that the exercise of control entails' (Bandura, 1982 p.142). In so doing, they may settle for 'proxy control' by entrusting another person with power (e.g. doctor, health visitor) to act on their behalf.

When considering self-efficacy, Bandura (1977b) suggests that an important distinction is made between perceived self-efficacy and expectation of the outcome. Perceived self-efficacy refers to people's judgements of their capabilities to execute given levels of performance, whilst expectation of the outcome are judgements of the likely consequences that such behaviour will produce. This may refer, for example, to a client's belief that following immunization a child will be protected from infectious disease, but if the client's perceived self-efficacy in actually presenting the child for what she feels is also a painful and even potentially hazardous procedure is low, then the benefits of taking the action will be overidden and the behaviour not performed.

The construct of self-efficacy has been subject to considerable empirical research in relation to its reliability in predicting and explaining health-related behaviour. O'Leary (1985) has published a comprehensive review of the literature in this area, covering such behaviour as cessation of smoking, eating disorders, pain experience and adherence to medical treatment. In relation to cessation of smoking, for example, O'Leary cites studies which have measured perceived self-efficacy at different stages of the process of giving up. McIntyre *et al.* (1983), for example, found that self-efficacy scores following behaviourial treatment for cessation of smoking were significant at three months and six months follow-up, and Colleti *et al.* (1981) found significant correlation between smoking rate and self-efficacy at three months follow-up. DiClemente (1986) found that perceived self-efficacy of clients who had stopped smoking after five months were significantly higher than those who had relapsed. O'Leary suggests that:

'these studies, in addition to demonstrating the predictive power of self-efficacy regarding smoking outcome, also suggest the potential utility of examining individuals' self-efficacy in order to tailor treatment to the needs of the individual'.

(O'Leary, 1985 p.440)

The nature of these studies suggests that perceived self-efficacy can be changed or enhanced, thus enabling an individual to feel more efficacious in carrying out a behaviour. Bandura (1977b) suggests a number of ways in which this could be achieved.

Performance accomplishment

This source of efficacy information is especially influential because it is based on personal mastery experiences. Successes raise mastery expectations; repeated failures lower them, particularly if the failures occur early in the course of events. After strong efficacy expectations are developed through repeated success, the negative impact of occasional failure is likely to be reduced. Thus, participant modelling or exposure may form the basis of the approach to a problem or behaviour which a client feels unable to cope with. For example, some success in breast-feeding may help a mother to overcome her uncertainty about it even if she has an occasional failure.

Vicarious experience

Bandura (1977b) also suggests that self-efficacy is influenced not only by personal experience, but also by observation of the experience of others. Thus, if another person is perceived to have mastery over a situation, then this could enhance the belief of the individual that she too could be successful. Following on with the breast-feeding example, a mother who has a low perceived self-efficacy may be helped by socializing with and observing other breast-feeding mothers.

Verbal persuasion

Bandura suggests that verbal persuasion is the most easily available technique for changing self-efficacy but not necessarily the most effective. Although an individual might be verbally persuaded that he can cope with an experience, these mastery expectations can be readily extinguished by discontinuing experiences. It is thought that the main value of social persuasion is in conjunction with performance mastery. In health visiting, the verbal contact is the practitioner's most readily available tool and must therefore be used with some caution if other techniques are not on offer.

Stress reduction

Stressful and taxing situations generally elicit emotional responses which, depending on the circumstances, might have informative value concerning personal competence. Therefore, emotional arousal is another source of information that can affect perceived self-efficacy. People rely partly on their state of psychological arousal in judging their anxiety and vulnerability to stress. Because high arousal usually inhibits performance, individuals are more likely to expect success when they are not beset by aversive stimuli than if they are tense and agitated. Thus, Bandura advocates that stress reduction should be attempted through helping people to develop mastery of aversive situations.

These four areas of influencing self-efficacy expectations clearly have implications for those involved with health-related behaviours, and particularly for assessing the desire and ability for client participation in health care. Steele *et al.* (1987) have suggested that self-efficacy provides a useful theoretical framework within which research can be conducted into patient participation and practice. They suggest that health professionals should assess their patients' self-efficacy perceptions and tailor interventions to those perceptions. The implications of this theory for the practice of health visiting is evident. Many situations faced by clients may be perceived to be stressful or taxing, for example, infant feeding, immunization or weight reduction. The evidence, as discussed by O'Leary (1985), appears to suggest that performance of these types of behaviour can be predicted by a person's perceived self-efficacy. It would seem that an understanding of the concept and its application is important if health visitors are to enable clients to feel more in control of their health. As

Steele *et al.* (1987) have proposed:

'Clinicians should therefore actively elicit and try to understand their patients' perspectives and formulate approaches to treatment that are in line with those perspectives'.

(p.20)

Taking the self-efficacy theory to its logical conclusion, this may include acceptance that a client's perceived self-efficacy is too low to carry out a behaviour. This may mean working through an experience with them or giving them opportunities to observe others successfully carrying out the behaviour, in conjunction with some verbal encouragement and anxiety reduction measures.

Relevance to health visiting and rationale for the theory

Bandura's theory seems particularly pertinent to health visiting from two perspectives. Firstly, existing research into health visiting has found that the role of the health visitor is often perceived by clients as being one of support, in which the professional is helping the client to cope with stressful life events, particularly the experience of child birth and child rearing. For example, Orr (1978) in a study of women in Northern Ireland, found that they were generally positive towards their health visitor, perceiving her as a 'friend' or supportive agent. Other studies such as Foxman *et al.* (1982) and Mayall and Grossmith (1985) have also found that parents identify the role of the health visitor as being a helping one. Foxman's study, like that of Graham (1979), found this to be related to particular events such as breast-feeding. In the current research by the author (Kendall, in progress) it was found that of 75 mothers interviewed, 33 per cent expected to receive some sort of reassurance from the health visitor. However, some studies have shown that health visitors fail to meet this need among parents. For example, Ashley (1987) found that mothers perceived their health visitor to be exclusively concerned with the child's health and that they could not approach her with their own problems. In a sample of mothers, MacIntosh (1986) found that 'a very large proportion continued to see health visiting as being concerned with various forms of surveillance and control' and that only a minority recognized the supportive function. Nevertheless, mothers in many of the studies cited do report that aspects of bringing up children such as infant feeding, sleep and behaviour are stressful, especially with a first baby. These research findings suggest that in order to meet the needs and expectations of parents and in so doing help the parents to meet the health needs of their children, health visitors need a framework for assessment which will take into account the concept of coping and its relationship to health behaviour towards children. Bandura's theory includes coping as one of its major concepts and sees coping with stress and health behaviour to be intimately related to the individual's perceived self-efficacy. An assessment based on the mother's ability to cope with a situation, as seen from her own perspective, could enhance the health visitor's effectiveness in enabling the parent to achieve her child's health potential. Other models for health visiting in relation to stress have been suggested, notably Clark's (1985) interpretation of the Neuman (1972) model of nursing, which is derived from system's theory. Clark proposes that the family can be seen as an open system, the integrity of which is maintained by the prevention or reduction of stress. The role of the health visitor is to identify and prevent such stress destabilizing the system. The problem with this approach is the undeniable fact that the theory is based in engineering science, where systems can never be more than the sum of their parts. A holistic approach to nursing or health visiting would suggest that the behaviours and responses of an individual or family are more complex than the sum of their parts. For example, primary prevention of infectious diseases through immunization is rarely a simple equation of educating parents and the necessary action being taken as a result. Research by Perkins (1982) has shown the complex decision-making process that parents go through prior to having their child immunized. This is related to their fears and beliefs about the effects of the injection as well as factors such as access to clinics and information. Assess-

ment of need therefore requires an approach which takes account of the health of family members within their social, psychological and biological context and from the perspective of the client. Bandura's theory appears to provide such a framework. The second area of research and debate which provides a rationale for applying Bandura's work is the increasing interest in clients participating as equal partners in their health care. A Health Visitors' Association (HVA) document (1988) has addressed the need for clients to be more involved in the process of planning and executing their care:

'Health visitors and school nurses must actively pursue the breaking down of barriers in professional/client relationships and act as facilitators to enable clients to participate in their own health care'.

(p.27)

This argument is based on research and discussion which suggests that clients are more satisfied with the care they receive and more likely to carry out healthy behaviour if they have participated in the process. For example, Roter (1977) found that when patients were given opportunities to ask questions about their treatment, they were more likely to comply. Ross (1988) found that information sharing about drug regimes with elderly people increased their understanding and knowledge of the treatment and also knowledge within the primary health care team. There is also a social trend towards a more consumer-orientated society where the client no longer wishes to be told what to do but to be a participant in decision-making. Sociologists such as Zola (1972) have described health professionals as agents of social control. In order to move away from this position, which is still apparent in studies of practice such as those by MacIntosh (1986) and Mayall and Foster (1988), health visitors have to adopt an approach which takes the client's perspective into account. The HVA have recognized this need for change in a paper entitled 'Whither Health Visiting?' (Goodwin, 1988). Under the heading 'imperatives for change' one finds:

'An increasing emphasis upon active user participation in health care and a more equal partnership between health visitor and client.'

(p.6)

Bandura's theory offers a framework in which client participation can preside because it takes as its starting point the perceived self-efficacy of the client. If the health visitor is able to assess the extent to which a parent feels able to cope with a situation and take action, then care planning will, of necessity, start from the client's point of view rather than that of the health visitor, whose own perceptions of the situation might be very different. As Steele *et al.* (1987) suggest, whilst a client may find herself overwhelmed by a particular problem, helping her to increase her self-efficacy through one of the methods suggested by Bandura may increase her participation in the process of planning care and her ability to cope.

Assessment of the Harris family using Bandura's theory of self-efficacy

When the health visitor visited Dawn Harris her primary objectives, as already stated, were to discuss the start of the immunization programme for Jamie and to introduce the topic of weaning him onto solid foods. The health visitor was concerned that Jamie had not yet had his first immunization, especially as Dawn had rigorously kept appointments with Michael, and the health visitor was aware that two appointments had been sent to Dawn over the last three months. As she had not seen Dawn and the children in the clinic she made an appointment to visit their home.

Bearing Bandura's framework in mind, the health visitor assessed the situation she observed in the family according to four broad questions:

- What are the needs or problems as Dawn perceives them?
- How does Dawn perceive her emotional response to the problem?

- What are Dawn's outcome expectations of any given behaviour?
- To what extent does Dawn perceive herself able to cope (self-efficacy)?

Then in the process of planning care the question is:

- What measures can be taken to increase Dawn's perceived self-efficacy?

Whilst these broad headings helped the health visitor to structure her assessment, they also enabled her to ensure that planning future care was firmly based on Dawn's perception of her situation. The assessment is shown in Figure 2.1.

From the assessment, it is clear that the health visitor has tried to assess the family situation from the client's perspective. Although the health visitor's primary objectives were to discuss immunization and weaning, by using the concepts involved in Bandura's theory she has managed to establish not only how the client perceives her needs but also how she feels able to cope with them – her perceived self-efficacy. So although Dawn appears to be aware of the need for Jamie's immunization and diet, her feelings of inadequacy in what she feels should be routine baby care appear to stem from a lack of support. Using the client's own language in the assessment helps to clarify the situation as she perceives it. This in turn means that the care plan will be designed with the client in order to meet the needs as she perceives them. In Dawn's case the overall needs are threefold – her own need for more support and reassurance from her husband, the need to promote Michael's well-being through understanding and modifying his behaviour, and the need to promote and maintain Jamie's health through protective measures. The care plan designed to meet these needs using the approaches suggested by Bandura for increasing self-efficacy is shown in Figure 2.2. In order to formulate and to put this care plan into operation, the health visitor had to be both familiar with the concept of self-efficacy and with the approaches that Bandura suggests will help to increase a person's self-efficacy. So, for example, this health visitor rec-

Perceived needs/problems	Emotional response	Outcome expectations	Perceived self-efficacy
Husband is working excessive hours.	Fatigue, 'fed-up', lonely.	To be able to discuss feelings with Trevor and reach a compromise.	Both partners are too tense to have a sensible discussion. 'We end up rowing'.
Michael is being naughty: waking at night, bedwetting and has tried to hurt the baby.	Anger, guilt and worry that he will hurt Jamie.	To get Michael back into the 'nice little boy' that he was.	Feels too tired and cross to give Michael the attention, 'I just smack him if he wets the bed'.
Not managing the baby as well as Michael was managed: missed clinic appointments, having difficulty in organizing time to reach clinic on public transport and feels muddled about weaning. 'I've forgotten what I did with Michael.'	Inadequacy and out of control.	To be able to manage and cope with 'routine' baby care.	'Sometimes I'm on top of it, other times I need more support.'

Figure 2.1   Assessment of need using Bandura's theory of self-efficacy.

ognized two areas where attending a mother's group might be helpful and this was based on:

- Recognizing Dawn's perceived needs to reduce stress through relaxation and companionship.
- Understanding that self-efficacy could be increased by reducing aversive stimuli.
- Recognizing that a group with women in a similar position could provide both a relaxing experience and the opportunity for Dawn to observe the behaviour of others (vicarious experience).

Thus the care plan was based firmly within a theoretical framework for action which provides the structure and rationale for practice. Because the concept of self-efficacy is so inherently linked to client participation, the care plan could not be formulated without consultation with Dawn on an equal basis. The framework also provided the structure for ensuring that the health of the children was not isolated from the family context. The

health visitor recognized that her own goals of immunization and weaning were not going to be achieved whilst Dawn was at a stage where she felt unable to cope with some aspects of her family life. It was therefore necessary to approach the problems systematically in the priority order that Dawn perceived them. An underlying problem was obviously one of communication between Dawn and Trevor, and this needed to be addressed before Dawn's self-efficacy in coping with her children's health could be increased.

The evaluation criteria were also worked out in partnership. This means that the criteria were in line with Dawn's outcome expectations as outlined in the assessment (Figure 2.1). In order for a care plan to be effective, the client has to feel that the goals are realistic, the action is within her capabilities and the evaluation of any action is acceptable to herself. Such an approach could enable the client to feel in control of the health of herself and her family and also enhance the role of the health visitor as a facilitator rather than a 'busybody'.

Need/problem	Aim	Action	Evaluation criteria
Tension between partners leading to inability to discuss Dawn's need for more support at home and companionship.	To reduce tension in the family so that Dawn feels more able to cope.	*Verbal persuasion* Talk to Dawn about how she could be efficacious in approaching Trevor. Encourage her to find out what his feelings are and to take them into account.	Dawn and Trevor will be able to have a reasoned discussion enabling them to reach a compromise on the amount of time Trevor spends at work e.g. one evening a week will be spent with the family.
		Stress reduction Explore with Dawn methods of reducing stress/anxiety e.g. join a mother's group to reduce isolation or recommend relaxation techniques.	Dawn will feel less isolated and more relaxed.
Behavioural difficulties in Michael leading to Dawn feeling angry/guilty and sometimes expressing this physically. Dawn needs to understand more about why Michael is expressing himself in this way.	To help Dawn to understand Michael's behaviour so that he can feel a valued family member.	*Verbal persuasion* Encourage Dawn to look at the family from Michael's point of view and how her response to him is currently reinforcing his behaviour. Give her *information* about the needs of a young child trying to cope with a new baby.	Dawn will feel more able to appreciate Michael's needs and her self-efficacy perception will increase. Michael will respond more positively to Jamie.
		Vicarious experience Dawn encouraged to join a mother's group where she will be able to share experience of bringing up a toddler and observe other people's coping strategies.	Dawn's self-efficacy will further be reinforced.
		Personal mastery Give Dawn practical advice on management of sleep problem and bed-wetting e.g. Michael to keep a chart on number of nights with a dry bed and award stars and small token prize for three stars etc.	Michael will be dry at night for at least five nights in the next two weeks. He will also sleep more regularly.
Jamie is behind in commencement of primary immunization and weaning is haphazard. Dawn feels unable to manage.	To enable Dawn to feel more in control of organizing her management of the children so that protective health activities are carried out e.g. daily routine including meal times. To set realistic dates to attend local clinic.	*Personal mastery* Remind Dawn of how she was able to maintain control over Michael's babyhood and explore the different perspectives. Arrange for Dawn to attend a more local clinic so that she feels in control of achieving the aim. Give Dawn further *information* about weaning so that will feel less confused.	Dawn will feel she is in control. Jamie will commence immunization and weaning process will be understood by Dawn and carried out.

Figure 2.2 Care plan using Bandura's theory of self-efficacy.

Evaluation and critique of the theory

Clearly, in order to make use of the concept of self-efficacy, the health visitor needs to have developed considerable communication skills to be able to ask the appropriate questions and to be able to listen to the client and make sense of the perspective she is offering. This is an area which few researchers in the field of self-efficacy have addressed. Bandura offers the theory as an explanation of people's behaviour, but he offers very little advice on how it should be applied in practice. Steele *et al.* (1987), whilst advocating its use in practice and suggesting that practitioners should 'elicit' their clients' perceived self-efficacy, give no guidance as to how this should be achieved.

Some studies have addressed the issue of measuring self-efficacy. A report by Weitzel (1989), for example, has demonstrated the important predictive power of perceived self-efficacy on health promotion behaviour among blue collar workers. Self-efficacy in this study was measured using a scale developed by Sherer *et al.* (1982). The scale consists of a 17 item Liker-type instrument with scores ranging from 17 to 85, the higher scores indicating higher self-efficacy. Whilst this approach is appropriate for research purposes, it does not readily lend itself to a practice situation where it would be inappropriate to expect clients to complete a questionnaire. This is particularly true in a profession such as health visiting, where clients' needs are very diverse and the role of the practitioner is very broad. It would appear, then, that health visitors do need to address their communication style if they are to use self-efficacy as a conceptual framework for practice. Research to date in this area demonstrates that there is increasing interest in examining the process of health visitor/client interaction, but that interpretations are conflicting. Warner (1984) reported that health visitors were skilled in their interactions with clients because, she claimed, goals were achieved. However, the evidence she presents suggests that the goals set were those of the health visitor and not goals determined in consultation with the client. Montgomery–Robinson (1986) reports a similar

degree of skill in the achievement of objectives by health visitors but again fails to acknowledge the client's perspective. Conversely, Sefi (1985) found that health visitors tended to rely on an interrogative approach with emphasis on advice-giving which belied the clients' perceived needs. Current research by the author (Kendall, in progress) corroborates this finding. The study provides evidence that health visitors' and clients' perceptions of a visit frequently differ and that the health visitor/client interaction can explain, to some extent, why this is so. The evidence appears to suggest that health visitors often have an agenda for visiting which they are reluctant to abandon regardless of the cues that clients might be providing about their own perception of the situation. With reference to the theoretical framework under discussion here, the implications are that health visitors need to change their approach in line with HVA recommendations (1988) in order to take on a more client centred attitude. Furthermore, communication skills training should occupy a much greater part in the curriculum than is currently the case. Given the skills to question sensitively, listen and facilitate client participation, self-efficacy could be usefully employed as a conceptual approach to practice.

However, another problem that arises from Bandura's presentation of self-efficacy and the research studies cited which have attempted to validate the theory, is the concept of behaviour change. It can be argued that there are ethical problems involved in trying to manipulate the behaviour of others, no matter how well-intentioned this may be. This is an issue that Bandura does not address. He assumes that if a person is unable to cope with a particular behaviour then it is right to increase that person's self-efficacy through a variety of measures which reduce aversive stimuli, and thereby induce a psychological change towards the desired behaviour. The question of ethics is pertinent to all health promotion activities, and indeed as Seedhouse (1988) points out, there are very few situations in health care which do not demand some attention to the moral dimension. The question of whether it is right to try and change a person's perceived self-efficacy may depend on the ethical stance adopted by the health visitor. For example, a deontological approach would demand that it is the duty of the health visitor to protect the child at any cost, whilst a utilitarian practitioner would take the view that the outcome for the whole family is more important than a perceived duty. The health visitor may not be conscious of the 'label' applied to her own moral philosophy but clearly it is important that practitioners address these issues when applying a theoretical framework to their practice.

In conclusion, it would seem that Bandura's theory of self-efficacy does offer a conceptual framework to the health visitor which provides a structure in which to practice from the client's perspective. Whilst the concept of self-efficacy itself may not be familiar to health visitors, the majority will have experienced situations where children cannot reach their full health potential because the parents are finding aspects of family life difficult to cope with. Bandura's theory offers both an explanation for the inability to change or adapt behaviour and guidance as to how self-efficacy can be increased. However, there are problems associated with the level of communication skills required to operate the theory and possible ethical dilemmas surrounding the notion of psychological manipulation which health visitors would need to address. The theory needs further testing as a conceptual framework for practice within all aspects of nursing care but particularly in the field of prevention and health promotion, where the concept of client participation is paramount in the future development of the role of the health visitor and child health in the community.

References

Ashley Y (1987). *Do health visitors really understand women's needs?* Paper given at the International Primary Health Care Conference, Westminster, September 1987.

Bandura A (1977a). *Social Learning Theory*. Prentice Hall, Englewood Cliffs, New Jersey.

Bandura A (1977b). Self-efficacy: Towards a theory of behaviourial change. *Psychological Review*; **84(2)**: 191–215.

Bandura A (1982). Self-efficacy mechanism in human agency. *American Psychology*; **37**: 122–47.

Barker W (1984). *Child Development Programme*. Early Childhood Development Unit, Senate House, University of Bristol.

Bedford H (1988). The importance of professional advice in achieving high immunization uptake. *Health Visitor*, **61(9)**: 286–7.

Clark J (1973) *A Family Visitor*. Royal College of Nursing, London.

Clark J (1985). *The Process of Health Visiting*. Unpublished PhD thesis, Polytechnic of the South Bank, London.

Colletti G, Supnick J and Rizzo A (1981). *An analysis of relapse determinants of treated smokers*. Paper presented at the meeting of the American Psychological Association, Los Angeles. Cited by O'Leary A (1985).

DiClemente C (1986). Self-efficacy and the addictive behaviours. *Journal of Social and Clinical Psychology*; **4**: 302–15.

Foxman R, Moss P, Boland G *et al.* (1982). A consumer view of the health visitor at six weeks post-partum. *Health Visitor*, **55(6)**: 302–5, 308.

Goodwin S (1988). *Whither Health Visiting?* Health Visitors' Association, London.

Graham H (1979). Women's attitudes to the child health services. *Health Visitor*, **52**: 175–8.

Health Visitors' Association (1988). *Bridging the Gap*. HVA, London.

Kendall S (in progress). *An Analysis of the Health Visitor/Client Interaction*. Ph.D. thesis, King's College, University of London.

Mayall B and Grossmith C (1985). The health visitor and the provision of services. *Health Visitor*, **58(12)**: 349–52.

Mayall B and Foster M–C (1988). *Parents and health visitors: Perspectives on preventive health care*. Thomas Coram Research Unit, London.

MacIntosh J (1986). *A Consumer Perspective on the Health Visiting Service*. Social and Paediatric Research Unit, University of Glasgow.

McIntyre K, Lichenstein E and Mermelstein R (1983). Self-efficacy and relapse in smoking cessation: a replication and extension. *Journal of Consulting Clinical Psychology*; **51**: 632–3.

Montgomery–Robinson K (1986). Accounts of health visiting, in While A (ed), *Research in Preventive Community Nursing Care*, John Wiley, Chichester.

Neuman B and Young R (1972). A model for teaching total person approach to patient problems. *Nursing Research*; **21(3)**: 264–9.

O'Leary A (1985). Self-efficacy and health. *Behaviourial Research Therapy*; **23(4)**: 437–45.

Orr J (1978). *Consumer Perspectives on Health Visiting*, Unpublished MSc thesis, University of Manchester.

Perkins E (1982). *Decision-making: The whooping cough dilemma*. Leverhulme practical papers in health education, No.8, University of Nottingham.

Ross F (1988). Information sharing between patients, nurses and doctors: Evaluation of a drug guide for old people in primary health care, in Johnson R (ed), *Recent Advances in Nursing: Excellence in Nursing*, vol. 21. Churchill Livingstone, Edinburgh.

Roter D (1977). Patient participation in the patient-provider interaction: The effect of patient question asking on the quality of interaction, satisfaction and compliance. *Health Education Monographs*; **5(4)**: 281–315.

Seedhouse D (1988). *Ethics – the Heart of Health Care*. John Wiley, Chichester.

Sefi S (1985). *The First Visit: A Study of Health Visitor/Mother Verbal Interactions*. Unpublished MA Dissertation, University of Warwick.

Sherer M, Maddox J, Mercandante B *et al.* (1982). The self-efficacy scale: construction and validation. *Psychological*

Reports; **51**: 663–71.

Steele D, Blackwell B, Gutmann M *et al.* (1987). The activated patient: dogma, dream or desideratum? *Patient Education and Counselling*, **10**: 3–23.

Warner U (1984). Asking the right questions. *Nursing Times,* *Community Outlook*; **13 June**: 214–6.

Weitzel M (1989). A test of the health promotion model with blue collar workers. *Nursing Research*; **38(2)**: 99–104.

Zola I (1972). Medicine as an institution of social control. *Sociological Review*; **20(4)**: 487–509.

3

Caring for a neonate in hospital using Roy's adaptation model
Hazel Mackenzie

The neonate in hospital – Roy's model applied

The purpose of this chapter is to examine some of the problems posed by the admission of a very young infant to hospital and to review, apply and evaluate Roy's adaptation model as a framework for delivering care. The discussion begins with an overview of some research related to the neonate and his family as a basis for outlining some of the priorities for care, followed by presentation of a case history to which the model can be applied.

The next section will provide an outline of Roy's model and the rationale for its selection, followed by application of the model to the admission of the three-week-old-infant, including nursing assessment and care plan. The concluding section will provide an evaluation of the model in this setting and overall critique of the tool as a nursing model.

Overview of research

The neonate

In the past it has been thought, and indeed may well have been convenient to think, that the neonate was a passive individual unable to react to, affect, or be affected by his environment. The research by Schaffer (1982), Bower (1977) and many others showing that this is clearly not the case, has important implications for those working in the neonatal setting.

The psychologist Piaget had a major influence on current views of the development of reason, perception, language and thought in the child. He saw the child as being cognitively active and inventive, continually striving to construct an understanding of events in his world in order to make sense of the environment. Piaget assumed that the purpose of knowledge was to enable the individual to adapt to the world in which they live (Piaget, 1972).

Piaget's stage theory of development suggests that during the sensorimotor stage, from birth to two years, children explore their environment through their senses and gradually assimilate new information and produce modified behaviour to accommodate new experiences in a highly sophisticated fashion.

Many nurses and parents still believe that neonates, like rats or kittens, are blind at birth. However, there is evidence to suggest that the neonate has vision not only at birth but in the last three months of pregnancy when there is sensitivity to light, although this is largely understimulated unless the mother sunbathes (MacFarlane, 1977).

In the enface position the neonate can engage in mutual eye contact with another person. The focal length is more or less fixed at 8–10 inches and this corresponds well with the distance between infant and carer's face during feeding. The mutual eye-gazing encourages the care-giver to talk to the baby and at three to six weeks the baby will respond to this with a smile (Bower, 1977). Lipsitt (1977) suggests that the neonate will search for a human face, which is preferred to other stimulation. A preference is also shown for bright and slow moving objects.

Auditory stimulation, like visual stimulation can be highly important. Again MacFarlane (1977) suggests that the fetus can respond to sound, indicating the presence of hearing. After birth, sounds are muffled for a few days until amniotic fluid is absorbed from the ear, after which neonates can locate sounds by turning and looking towards the source. Furthermore, Condon and Sander (1974) and Bower (1977), amongst other researchers, have found that neonates move their arms and legs in synchronous rhythm to the sound of their parents' speech.

As well as visual and auditory stimulation, the neonate is very sensitive to touch. Wolff (1969) made some interesting observations on the distress demonstrated by three-day-old babies in response to nakedness. Regardless of environmental temperature, they were only comforted by swaddling. Klaus and Faranoff (1979) found that high risk neonates nursed on sheepskins, rocked and cuddled, gained weight and developed faster than controls. While Kramer and Pierport (1976) found that neonates stimulated with rocking and tape recordings of a woman's voice and heartbeat also gained weight at a faster rate than controls.

The concept of stimulation brings to focus the now topical issue of pain in the neonate. Roberts (1988) comments on the glaring omission of this topic from textbooks, suggesting that many writers still regard the neonate as insensitive to pain, while Owens (1986) suggest that more accurate methods of pain assessment must be sought in an attempt to find safe ways to alleviate it.

Bonding

Any discussion on the neonate in or out of hospital cannot proceed for long without addressing the controversial issue of bonding. In 1950, John Bowlby took up an appointment with the World Health Organization to look at the psychological aspects of children who were orphaned or separated from the families and in need of care in an institution or foster home. As a result of his findings Bowlby states that:

'among the most significant developments in psychiatry in the last quarter century has been the steady growth of evidence that the quality of the parental care which a child receives in his earliest years is of vital importance to his future mental health.'

(Bowlby, 1965, p.13)

Bowlby felt that what is essential for mental health is that an infant or young child should experience a warm, intimate and continuous relationship with his mother or permanent mother substitute. Bowlby supported his rather dramatic conclusion with numerous follow-up and retrospective studies demonstrating that groups of children separated from their parents in early years grew up with a high incidence of teenage delinquency and he stated that:

'there is a very strong case indeed for believing that prolonged separation stands foremost amongst the causes of delinquent character formation.'

(Bowlby, 1965, p.41)

In 1972 Rutter produced a book entitled *Maternal Deprivation Reassessed* in which much of Bowlby's work is supported. However, Rutter does question the exclusiveness of the mother–child relationship, stating that:

'providing that those giving care remain constant in the child's early life, then multiple mothering need have no adverse effects.'

(p.25)

Klaus and Kennell (1976) introduced another facet into bonding and attachment theory by suggesting the existence of a sensitive period, during which the intimate mother–child contact gives rise to a cascade of reciprocal interactions which locks them together and mediates the further development of attachment. Klaus and Kennell go further to suggest that if a mother and child are separated during this time – which is thought to last from some hours to a day – then bonding will become impaired and even completely prevented.

If accepted at face value, the suggestions of these researchers have important implications for nurses, midwives and doctors working with neonates and their parents, particularly in cases where separation may be unavoidable. However, in the light of more recent research the work of Bowlby, Rutter, Klaus and Kennell has been heavily criticised.

Sluckin *et al.* (1983) state that every so often a psychological theory escapes the confines of sober academic debate and enters the wide public arena by way of publicity in the mass media. They further suggest that misguided ideas about mothering held by some nurses has led, in some cases, to harassment of those mothers who in the early stages appear to have difficulty relating to their babies.

'Liberalizing ideas in the field of child care and elsewhere can become oppressive when elevated into prescriptive dogmas.'

(p.18)

Richards (1984) states that early studies often suffer from serious methodological weakness, failing to take into account other influencing factors such as environment and experiences and the difficulties in measuring the phenomenon. Leiderman (1981) carried out follow-up studies of neonates separated in intensive care and concluded that the separated mothers and babies formed social bonds that could not be differentiated from bonds established by mothers and babies who had not been separated.

Tulman's research (1985) compared the pattern of newborn handling by 36 newly delivered primagravid mothers with 36 female nursing students on their first day in the newborn nursery. Tulman demonstrated significant differences between the two groups, both in the time spent handling and in the pattern of handling. The students demonstrated a pattern of using fingertips followed by palms, which Tulman suggested was a pattern evoked by a new situation. However, Klaus and Kennell in their work had used this very pattern of handling as an assessment of attachment between mothers and babies. Thus, another facet of the bonding dilemma is the reliability of methods of assessing bonding, which Tulman concludes, 'casts doubt on the validity of research findings supporting the theory of maternal–infant bonding' (p. 205).

While the benefits of Bowlby and other's work in instigating increased parental involvement and residency cannot be overlooked, the question of what are the implications of the bonding controversy for neonates, their parents and health professionals still remains.

The role of the father

It is interesting that in the work of Bowlby, Rutter and others very little mention is made of the father. Bowlby explains this by saying that almost all the evidence in his work concerns the relationship of child and mother 'which is without doubt in ordinary circumstances, by far the most important relationship during these years, the father's value being as the economic and emotional support of the mother' (Bowlby, 1965, p.16).

Pawson and Morris (1972) said of fathers:

'Unlike women they have no hormone changes, no remarkable physical and emotional experiences . . . it is a secondary form of relationship.'

(p.112)

Parke (1981) challenges these notions by suggesting that today no single type of father exists. Some remain uninvolved in child-rearing while others are active participants. However, social and economic changes have meant that, on the whole, fathers are more involved in child-rearing than in the past. Schaffer and Emerson (1964) found that by 18 months of age children were equally attached to their mothers and fathers, and they concluded that it was not the quantity of time fathers spent interacting with their children but the quality of that time. Power and Parke (1974) found that although mothers and fathers played the same games with their children they had clearly different styles, with fathers more often engaging in exploratory and 'rough and tumble' play.

In a review of research into fathering, Lamb (1973) suggests that mothers and fathers play different roles in their child's development: fathers

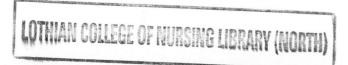

tend to provide more play and stimulation while mothers tend to provide comfort and nurturing care. The belief that the mother is the right person to give care is derived mostly from the fact that she typically does. It is therefore a cultural rather than biological influence.

Parental stress

Having looked at the relationships between the newborn and his family it now seems appropriate to examine some of the stresses on these relationships when a very young infant becomes sick.

The fact that parenthood can be regarded as a crisis in itself has been well documented. Cronenwett (1985) suggests that the crisis is viewed differently by mothers and fathers depending on the amount of role change involved. The crisis of parenthood can also be viewed differently between different sets of parents. The same can be said about parents' reactions to the infant's admission to hospital.

Smith et al. (1982) state that parents almost always experience anxiety. In severe anxiety a person's perceptual field narrows and what they hear and understand is distorted. Fear is also common, often exacerbated by inadequate information, while a feeling of powerlessness is common as parents lose the role of controller of their child's life, and become helpless, dependent and unsure of how to act. Parents may feel guilty – blaming themselves for their child's illness. When guilt is expressed Smith et al. (1982) suggest that it is often in the form of anger which may be directed towards the staff as convenient targets.

Jay (1977) observed that parents appeared immobile and unable to reach out to their sick child. Jay concluded that the greatest stress to parents of a sick child was role revision, which she described as 'giving up the role of parents of a well child and taking on the role of parents of a sick child' (p.150).

A study carried out by Riddle et al. (1987) looked at stress in an intensive care unit as perceived by parents and found significant differences between mothers' and fathers' perceptions of stress. Mothers rated the child's emotional behaviour as most stressful while fathers graded staff communi-cations as most stressful. The notion that mothers and fathers may perceive stressful situations differently is further supported by Mandell et al. (1980) who observed paternal responses to sudden unexplained infant death. In this study of 46 families, several mourning patterns seemed more characteristic of men. These were:

- an increase in business and workload;
- a feeling of reduced self-worth;
- self-blame due to lack of care involvement;
- marked inability to ask for help.

The studies reviewed here provide a brief outline of some of the research. Although not all the studies pertain directly to the very young infant, a number of important issues are apparent. Firstly, the vast amount of research on the complexity and sophistication of neonatal behaviour, along with the suggestion that stimulation or its lack can influence infant development, has important implications for nurses and doctors working with neonates and their parents. In the hospital setting, the sick young infant may well be nursed naked, exposed to noise, bright lights and painful procedures. The opportunity for pleasant stimulation, mutual eye gazing, touch and rocking may well be reduced. It follows that a priority of care must be the implementation of research findings to manipulate the environment and maximize the infant's development.

With regard to bonding, the nurse has a responsibility to examine research findings in greater depth than is provided here, and form her own opinions. In practice the nursing priority is to encourage parental involvement and residency where possible and assist the parents to meet the needs of their sick baby.

Research into fatherhood suggests that fathers can no longer be regarded as just a biological necessity. Infants need contact with their fathers just as the fathers need contact with their newborn babies. It is therefore another priority that paediatric nurses assess individual fathers and their role and refrain from merely paying lip-service to the notion of family-centred care.

Finally, parental stress may well be a normal and inevitable response when a baby is ill. However, the parental response to that stress will vary from parents to parents and requires individual assessment within each family to assist their adaptation to a new situation. The paediatric nurse has an important role in assessing the neonate, the mother and the family. Only then will she be embracing the true principles of family-centred care.

Presentation of the case

With these research priorities in mind, the case was selected in an attempt to test Roy's model as a nursing model for family-centred care. The special care or intensive care setting was deliberately not selected so as to avoid the tendency to concentrate on the neonate's physiological problems. Instead, the paediatric surgical ward setting was selected.

Tony was three weeks old and was the first child of Mr and Mrs Smith, a young married couple. Until the birth of Tony, Mrs Smith had been a primary school teacher while Mr Smith was an architect. Tony had been a well baby until the morning of admission.

In the early morning Mrs Smith had noticed that Tony appeared to be unsettled and in some pain. On changing his nappy a lump was noted in his right groin. Mrs Smith contacted her general practitioner who suggested that she should take Tony to the hospital.

In the accident and emergency department, both parents were seen by the senior registrar, who after examining Tony diagnosed an incarcerated inguinal hernia. Diamorphine was administered to Tony and the hernia was manually reduced.

Tony was admitted to the paediatric surgical ward. The medical instructions were to place Tony in gallows traction to maintain reduction of the hernia. The medical plan was to keep Tony as settled as possible to facilitate reduction or any swelling with a view to surgery in 24 hours to perform a right inguinal herniotomy.

On admission Tony appeared settled and sleepy after his diamorphine. Both Mr and Mrs Smith seemed anxious and worried. Mrs Smith in particular looked flushed and agitated. Both parents were aware of the medical plans but were keen to ask questions about the gallows traction about which they seemed unclear. Time was taken at this point to introduce staff members and answer some of the immediate questions that the parents had. Mr and Mrs Smith were introduced to another family on the ward whose baby was being nursed in gallows traction. This gave the Smith family time to settle into the ward and ask questions before the traction was applied. During this time Tony was peacefully asleep in his mother's arms, which both parents found reassuring following the stress of Tony's earlier discomfort and the rushed journey to hospital.

Roy's adaptation model – outline and rationale for selection

After considering the case presented, it was decided to select Roy's adaptation model as a basis for formulating a family-centred care plan. The full rationale for its selection will be discussed after outlining the elements of the model.

Roy's model draws from the work of Harry Helson (1964), a physiological psychologist, who developed the theory of adaptation from work in the field of visual perception, and focused on the adaptation of rods and cones in the eye in response to light. The Roy's adaptation model can be viewed primarily as a systems model. Man is regarded as a system, divided into subsystems and influenced by stimuli in both his internal and external environment. When faced with stimuli the person must adapt; in health terms failure to adapt positively results in ill health (Figure 3.1).

If we accept that a nursing model is intended to describe the reality of patient care and guide our nursing practice, then a well-constructed model should contain the following information:

- some basic assumptions on the nature of the person receiving care;
- the cause of the problem requiring nursing intervention;
- the nature of assessment;
- the goals for nursing intervention;

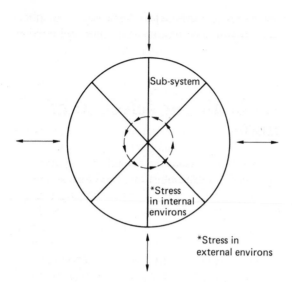

Figure 3.1   The dynamics of a systems model.

- knowledge and skills required for care;
- a statement on the function of the nurse;
- the nature of evaluation.

In simple terms:

- Who is the recipient of care?
- What is the nature of the care?
- When is care required?
- How is that care delivered?

Basic assumptions

Roy is very clear on what she regards as eight basic assumptions on the nature of the person requiring care. An appreciation of these assumptions is essential to the understanding of the model (Roy, 1980).

- The person is a biopsychosocial being.
- The person is in constant interaction with a changing environment.
- To cope with a changing world the person uses both innate and acquired mechanisms which are biological, psychological and social in origin.
- Health and illness are one inevitable dimension of person's life.

- To respond positively to environmental changes the person must adapt.
- The person's adaptation is a result of the stimuli he is exposed to and his own adaptation level. Stimuli can be divided into:
    Focal – factors immediately confronting the person.
    Contextual – other factors in the environment.
    Residual – beliefs, attitudes and previous experience.
- The person's adaptation level is such that it comprises a 'zone' indicating the range of stimulation that will lead to a positive response.
- The person is perceived as having four modes of adaptation.
    Physiological needs – associated with body structure and function.
    Self-concept – the way a person perceives himself.
    Role-function – psychosocial unity and social expectations.
    Interdependence – the balance between independence and dependence.

Cause of problems requiring intervention

From Roy's assumptions it would appear that the cause of problems likely to require nursing intervention are as follows. When a person is faced with a stimulus he must adapt in response to that stimulus in order to maintain equilibrium. Failure to adapt leads to maladaption. Therefore, nursing intervention is required when a person demonstrates maladaptive behaviour in response to a stimulus or when that stimulus falls outside the person's adaptation zone.

Nature of assessment

According to Roy's model the aim of assessment is two-fold. The first level assessment is aimed at identifying behaviour which is maladaptive or inappropriate. When behaviour has been identified as maladaptive, the nurse moves to the second level assessment which is aimed at identifying stimuli or influencing factors in the environment that have caused the maladaptive behaviour. These stimuli may be focal, contextual or residual. The four modes of adaptation – physical needs, self-concept, role function and interdependence – provide a framework for assessment, ensuring that no area of the individual's behaviour is omitted. Following the two level assessment, patient problems, both actual and potential, are identified.

Goals for nursing intervention

In Roy's theory the goal for nursing intervention is to assist the individual to adapt to presenting stimuli in a positive way, thus freeing energy to respond to other stimuli in the environment. If adaptation is already positive, then the goal for care is to assist the individual in maximizing and maintaining strategies for coping. Goals should be related to achieving adaptive responses in all modes, stated in behavioural terms, guided by a knowledge of norms and planned in conjunction with the patient.

Knowledge of skills required for care

To facilitate adaptation it is necessary for the nurse to have knowledge of all four modes of adaptation and an ability to recognize adaptive and maladaptive behaviour in each mode. An understanding of the ranges of behaviour which are acceptable as normal is required, along with an appreciation of the stresses which can affect behaviour and methods of altering stimuli to promote adaptation.

The function of the nurse

According to Roy the unique function of the nurse is to focus 'on the patient as a person adapting to these stimuli present as a result of his position on the health-illness continuum' (Roy, 1980, p.263).

The nature of evaluation

Evaluation of care involves a reassessment of the patient in all four modes, to assess whether or not the patient is now demonstrating a positive response and to aim the nursing care at maintaining

that response. If maladaptive behaviour is identified then goals for care require to be reset and nursing care reconsidered.

Rationale for selection of model

A number of reasons lie behind the selection of Roy's model for the assessment and formation of a care plan for the Smith family. Studying the research relating to the neonate and his family in conjunction with the case presented, the concept of adaptation seems pertinent not only to the neonate but the whole family. As previously discussed, the birth of a child, particularly the first child, requires much adaptation on the part of the parents. However, when that child becomes a sick child, in addition to pre-existing stress, then maladaptive behaviour is more likely.

Some alteration of the model has been necessary in that although it has been described by Roy in terms of 'the person' or 'his' it has been inferred that Roy's model can equally be applied as a family-centred model. The model's structure facilitates this application and is another basis for its selection in preference to other nursing models that are not easily applied to the family setting.

The concept of first and second level assessment incorporated in Roy's model is appealing because during the first level assessment maladaptive behaviour is identified, while the second level assessment identifies the influencing factors. Since nursing care is aimed at the manipulation of stimuli in the patient's environment, it is vital to identify these stimuli for goal setting and intervention. Thus nursing care should be given direction in this way and directed to the cause of the problem, rather than vaguely to the problem itself.

Finally, the separation of modes of adaptation into physiological needs, self-concept, role function and interdependence should ensure that nursing care is directed to all aspects of the family, and there should be no risk that the nursing model merges back into becoming a medical model for care. Furthermore, the four modes should assist in the assessment of different anxieties that parents present and avoid 'potential anxiety' as an umbrella term describing a variety of problems.

Roy's model applied – assessment and care plan

The proceeding section provides a nursing assessment and care plan for the Smith family carried out in the evening of admission to hospital. Tony was placed in gallows traction with his parents present and assisting. Mr Smith had to fly to London that evening for a business meeting, while Mrs Smith had decided to be resident in the hospital and accommodation had been arranged in the 'mother's unit'.

It is beyond the scope of this chapter to provide intra- and post-operative assessments, but it is felt that the assessment and care plan provided below will adequately demonstrate the application of Roy's model and provides sufficient discussion for its evaluation.

In keeping with Roy's intention, a two level assessment was carried out in the four modes of physiological, self-concept, role-function and interdependence, observing behaviour in each mode. During the first level assessment, behaviour was observed using the nurse's knowledge of normal, and maladaptive behaviour that caused concern was identified. During the second level assessment, influencing factors were considered in terms of focal, contextual and residual stimuli as a basis for directing care (Figure 3.2).

Following the assessment the care plan was formulated (Figure 3.3). Actual and potential problems were identified, expected outcomes were stated in terms of anticipated behaviour and nursing action was described.

Nursing intervention may be aimed at altering the stimuli in such a way that they fall within the family's existing adaptation level, such as supporting and demonstrating techniques of Tony's care in a way that enables the parents to master difficulties. Alternatively, nursing action may be aimed at extending the parents' adaptation level to cope with the stimuli – for example reducing anxiety by providing information, encouraging the parents to ask questions and offering support. Evaluation is not documented but, as previously stated, would involve a reassessment of the family and resetting of goals if appropriate or supporting the parents' positive adaptation.

Evaluation and critique of model

Aggleton and Chalmers (1984) suggest that nursing models should not be seen as good or bad, right or wrong. Rather, they should be seen as guidelines within which to explore the pertinence of particular approaches to care in different nursing contexts. Bearing in mind the previous rationale for selecting Roy's model, the concept of adaptation was found to be appropriate to the setting selected.

The division of assessment into two levels was useful as a guide to planning care, in that the care was directed to the 'root' cause of the problem. Furthermore it emphasized the individuality of responses to hospitalization such as anxiety, fear or guilt. Although the two level assessment was useful, there was some difficulty in determining the difference between focal, contextual and residual stimuli. On this point the model could benefit from further clarity.

The inclusion of the four modes of adaptation again gave structure to the assessment and was particularly useful in defining different parental anxieties. The physiological mode provided satisfactory guidance for this particular setting but may require development for application to a sicker child and family and may be difficult to apply to the intensive care setting where physiological problems alter rapidly. This suggestion is supported by Wagner (1976) and Roy (1976).

There was a certain amount of overlap between the different modes. In particular there was overlap between physiological and role function in connection with difficulty in breast-feeding Tony. Similarly between role function and interdependence in relation to demonstration of dependence on nursing staff and Mrs Smith's poor understanding of technical care and medical plan.

Since Roy (1970) suggests that man is simultaneously a biopsychosocial being, it is arguable that some overlap should be expected, is in fact

I Physiological	Behaviour	Focal	Contextual	Residual
Oxygen and circulation	No current difficulties noted. Colour good centrally and peripherally. Respiratory rate 32.			
Fluids and electrolytes	Tony appears well hydrated – good tissue turgor.			
Elimination	Tony wears disposable nappies. Has passed urine since admission – normal on ward testing. Normal breast-fed stool.			
Nutrition	Breast-fed on demand 3–4 hourly. Fed poorly at 12 midday and 3pm.	Tony is in gallows traction.	Mrs Smith found the position awkward for feeding.	Tony – received opiates this morning.
Rest and activity	Tony has been unsettled this afternoon.	Tony fed poorly.	Normally sleeps in the prone position.	Mrs Smith says that she normally carries Tony if he is unsettled.
Regulation	Tony's temperature is 36°C rectally.* Toes appear cold but are pink.	Legs are elevated and bandaged.	Tony is a small baby with a large surface area in relation to weight. The ward can be draughty.	

II Self-concept

	Behaviour	Focal	Contextual	Residual
Physical self	No problems observed for the family.			
Personal self	Both parents are upset at Tony's admission and surgery. They are particularly worried about 'the scar'.	Tony requires a right inguinal herniotomy.	Tony is 3/52 old and has never required hospitalization.	Parents have very little experience of hospitals.

III Role function

	Behaviour	Focal	Contextual	Residual
	Mrs Smith is concerned about her ability to breast-feed Tony. 'I'm really keen on breast-feeding, but maybe a bottle would be easier while he is in hospital.'	Tony is in a difficult position for breast-feeding.	Mrs Smith is now tired – the hospital environment provides little privacy compared with home.	Significant others have bottle-fed – Mrs Smith motivated to breast-feed.

IV Interdependence

	Behaviour	Focal	Contextual	Residual
	Both Mr and Mrs Smith are concerned about Tony's care on discharge.	Poor perception of Tony's surgery and future needs.	Emergency admission.	Parents have no previous experience of surgery.
	Mrs Smith has been asking the nurse caring for Tony to change his nappy. 'I don't think I can manage him in this position'.	Dependence on nurses. Tony's position is strange to Mrs Smith.	? Lack of confidence in parental role in hospital.	

Figure 3.2 Assessment of the Smith family.

* Eoff *et al.* (1974) noted the danger of rectal temperature measurement and found axillary temperature measurement both reliable and safe in infants. However, rectal temperature measurement continues to be used in neonatal care.

Problem	Desired outcome	Nursing action
A. Tony has been breast-feeding poorly this afternoon. Mrs Smith has found his position very awkward for feeding.	A feeding pattern that satisfies both Mrs Smith and Tony will be re-established.	– draw screens round family when feeding is in progress – offer encouragement to Mrs Smith to adopt different position – try lying on side in bed with Tony's face to the side *or* – try Mrs Smith sitting in the bed leaning over Tony in the enface position – chart feeding times on feed chart.

A.
Tony has been restless this afternoon
? due to pain
  hunger
  noise in the ward
  lack of pleasant tactile
    stimulation.
	Tony will appear more settled and sleep for longer periods.	– Mrs Smith is able to distinguish Tony's pain cry and hunger cry. She will guide the nurses as to analgesia requirements.
		– hernia site will be checked at nappy changes to ensure that it remains reduced
		– gallows traction will be maintained to encourage hernia to remain reduced
		– avoid unnecessary disturbance of Tony
		– Tony's bed will be placed in a quiet area of the ward
		– for comfort Tony will be nursed on a sheepskin
		– Mrs Smith plans to bring in some of Tony's musical toys and mobiles
		– encourage parents to touch Tony and stroke him when he is unsettled
		– check temperature per rectum 4 hourly.

A. Tony's toes are cold. **P.** Risk of constriction of circulation due to bandages.	Tony's toes will remain pink and warm.	– circulation checked hourly for colour, sensation, movement and warmth – bandages removed four hourly to check that Tony's skin is not marking – wrap Gamjee round Tony's legs – Mr Smith will bring in some booties.
A. Mr and Mrs Smith are worried about Tony's surgery. At present they have a poor understanding of what is involved.	Both parents will have a clear understanding of Tony's surgery and medical plan.	– liaise with medical staff with regard to treatment plans – reassure parents that Tony's admission should be for a few days only – discuss surgery with parents at a time when they are receptive to receiving information i.e. when Tony is more settled – reassure parents that they can accompany Tony to theatre and remain until he is asleep – discuss surgery using ward diagrams and care on return from theatre – describe position and expected size of scar

Figure 3.3 Care Plan for the Smith Family. (A = Actual; P = Potential)

Problem	Desired outcome	Nursing action
		– show Mr and Mrs Smith round the theatre suite – suggest that the parents write down any questions to ask the surgeon – introduce parents to Mr and Mrs Black whose baby Hailey (4 weeks old) had a left inguinal herniotomy today.
A. Mrs Smith is anxious about her maternal role in maintaining breast-feeding.	Mrs Smith will select the best method of feeding for Tony and herself.	– allocate the same staff member to family – continue to ease transition to new feeding position – reassure Mrs Smith that Tony will require to be in gallow's traction only until surgery is performed tomorrow – give support and encouragement verbally when feeding – reassure Mrs Smith that Tony appears well nourished.
A. Paternal role conflict due to meeting in London tomorrow.	Mr Smith will come to terms with a decision.	– support Mr Smith in whatever decision he comes to – if Mr Smith chooses to attend the meeting provide a hospital leaflet and telephone numbers, with names of nurses in charge – reassure Mr Smith that he can phone the ward at any time and as often as he wants to – provide privacy for parents to be together with Tony this evening.
A. Mrs Smith is demonstrating dependence on the nursing staff in meeting Tony's needs – due to difficulty with position in gallows traction and change in her normal routine.	Mrs Smith will demonstrate independence and confidence in caring for Tony.	– provide help requested by Mrs Smith – demonstrate changing of Tony's nappy and bandages – supervise Mrs Smith in changing nappy and bandages – show Mrs Smith where nappies and basins are stored in locker – encourage Mrs Smith to use her own babycare products and clothes – encourage Mrs Smith to hold and stimulate Tony as she would at home – encourage Mr Smith to continue his involvement with Tony.
A. Both parents are concerned about Tony's care on discharge.	Parents will be ready to care for Tony on discharge.	– liaise with medical staff about discharge – introduce parents to home care team tomorrow when they visit the ward – offer time for questions – provide information in discharge follow-up – be aware of the need to repeat this information again as necessary.

acceptable and does not detract from the quality of patient care. Furthermore, overlap from one mode to another with different emphasis on cause may enhance the care received by ensuring that all aspects of the problems are examined.

The model gives very little guidance on what constitutes adaptive or maladaptive behaviour and this appears to be very much a case of judgement based on the nurse's values. Thus, we run the risk of assuming that, for example, parental anxiety is an inevitable and normal behaviour on admission to hospital and therefore does not require nursing intervention.

On a finer point, Roy's model is based on adaptation theory and the identification of mal-adaptive behaviour. In a profession where there is active encouragement of the involvement of parents in care and of open discussion of our plans of care with them, the terms adaptive and maladaptive smack of delinquency and should be modified or omitted from the assessment form as illustrated.

There appears to be some disagreement over definitions and terminology in the literature on nursing models with words such as concept, theory and model being used almost interchangeably. Roy's original work was extremely difficult to follow due to the use of obscure language. This appears to be a common problem as Wright (1986) suggests, much of the writing on models has come from America and many of the theorists write in a style and language incomprehensible to most nurses. 'This can render valuable information inaccessible to "grassroots" nurses.'

There is a clear need for nursing theorists to avoid obscure and complicated language and to present their work in an intelligible fashion. Miller (1982) discusses the use of language in an article on the relationship between nursing theory and practice and concludes:

'if it is virtually impossible for experienced nurses to relate nursing theory to everyday nursing practice then something is very wrong with either the theory or the practice.'

(p.417)

The actual theoretical basis for Roy's model has come under attack from a variety of directions. The very fact that Roy bases her model on eight 'assumptions' suggests that the theory is open to further testing.

Many writers are critical of the application of general theory in nursing irrespective of the context in which it has been developed. McFarlane (1976) warns us to beware of clutching at any structural security which is not reflected in the reality of nursing practice.

Roy (1976) is quick to emphasize that the beliefs on which the model is based may not have been scientifically tested, or submitted to rigorous clinical research but have been accepted as true. Despite many modifications to the model, as late as 1980, Roy suggests that some of the assumptions should be validated and that there is potential for further clarification.

The debate over the theoretical content of nursing models is beyond the remit of this chapter; suffice to say that nursing theory requires to be research-based but also that nursing models need to be implemented. As early as 1968, Dicott wrote that theory is born of practice, it is refined in research and must and can be return to practice, if research is to be other than a draining of energy from the main business of nursing and theory more than idle speculation.

In conclusion, the use of Roy's adaptation model as a framework for planning care for Tony and his family had the advantage of providing structure for assessment and planning which ensured that not only the neonate's but the family's needs were considered in keeping with the initial priorities established. Certainly further development of the model is required, with more clarity in language use, but perhaps most important is that the model is implemented in nursing practice, since ultimately the best judge of a model is not the nurse but the patient.

References

Aggleton P and **Chalmers H** (1984). Models and theories – critical examination. *Nursing Times*; **81**(14): 38–9.
Bower TGR (1977). *The Perceptual World of the Child*. Fontana/Open Books, London.
Bowlby J (1965). *Child Care and the Growth of Love*. 2nd edition, Penguin, Harmondsworth, Middlesex.

Chapman CM (1985). *Theory of Nursing – Practical Application.* Harper and Row Publishers, London.

Condon W and Sander L (1974). Neonate movement synchronised with adult speech. Interactional participation and language acquisition. *Science*; 183: 99–101.

Cronenwett LR (1985). Parental network structure and perceived support after birth of first child. *Nursing Research*; 34(6): 347–52.

Dicott J (1986). Theory in a practice discipline. *Nursing Research*; 17(2): 415–35.

Eoff MJF, Meier RS and Miller C (1974). Temperature measurement in infants. *Nursing Research*; 23(6): 457–60.

Helson H (1964). *Adaptation Level Theory.* Harper and Row, New York.

Jay P (1977). Paediatric intensive care – involving parents in the care of their child. *Maternal Child Nursing Journal*; 2: 195–204.

Klaus MH and Fanaroff HB (1979). *Care of the High Risk Neonate.* 2nd edition. WB Saunders, Philadelphia.

Klaus MH and Kennell JH (1976). *Maternal-Infant Bonding.* Mosby Co, St Louis.

Kramer L and Pierpont M (1976). Rocking waterbeds and auditory stimulation to enhance growth of pre-term infants. *Journal of Pediatrics*; 99(2): 297–9.

Lamb ME (1973). *The Role of the Father in Child Development.* John Wiley, New York.

Leiderman PH (1981). Cited in Sluckin W, Herbert M and Sluckin A (1983). *Maternal Bonding.* Blackwell Publishers, New York.

Lipsitt LP (1977). The study of sensory and learning processes of the newborn. *Clinics in Perinatology*; 3(3): 163–87.

MacFarlane A (1977). *The Psychology of Childbirth.* Fontana/Open Books, London.

McFarlane JK (1976). The role of research and the development of nursing theory. *Journal of Advanced Nursing*; 1: 443–57.

Mandell F, McNaulty E, Reece R (1980). Observation of parental response to sudden unexplained infant death. *Pediatrics*; 65: 221–5.

Miller A (1982). The relationship between nursing theory and nursing practice. *Journal of Advanced Nursing*; 10: 417–24.

Owens ME (1986). A crying need. *American Journal of Nursing*; 86(1): 73.

Parke RD (1981). *Fathering.* Fontana Paperbacks, London.

Pawson M and Morris N (1972). *The Role of the Father in Pregnancy and Labour.* Karger, Basel.

Piaget J (1972). *The Child and Reality.* Penguin, Harmondsworth, Middlesex.

Power TC and Parke RD (1974). Play as a context for early learning, in Sigel IE and Laosa LM (eds), *The Family as a Learning Environment.* Plenum, New York.

Richards MPM (1984). The myth of bonding, in McFarlane JA (ed) *Progress in Child Health* vol. 1. Churchill Livingstone, Edinburgh. pp. 114.

Riddle JI, Hennessey J, Eberly TW *et al.*(1987). Stresses in the paediatric intensive care unit as perceived by mothers and fathers, in Barnes CM (ed), *Recent Advances in Nursing – Nursing Care of Children*; 16: 149–62. Longman Group UK, Ltd.

Roberts PM (1988). A cry for research – pain in the neonate. *Canadian Nurse*; 84(6): 17–9.

Roy C (1970). Adaptation – A conceptual framework for nursing. *Nursing Outlook*; 18(3): 42–5.

Roy C (1976). The Roy adaptation model – comment. *Nursing Outlook*; 24(11): 690–1.

Roy C (1980). The Roy adaptation model, in Rieh LJP and Roy C, *Conceptual Models for Nursing Practice* 2nd edition. Appleton-Century-Crofts, New York.

Rutter M (1972). *Maternal Deprivation Re-assessed.* Penguin, Harmondsworth, Middlesex.

Schaffer HR and Emerson PE (1964). The development of social attachments in infancy. *Monographs of Social Research in Child Development*; 29: 94.

Schaffer R (1982). *Mothering.* 4th edition, Fontana/Open Books, London.

Sluckin W, Herbert M and Sluckin A (1983). *Maternal Bonding.* Basil Blackwell Publishers, New York.

Smith MJ, Goodman JA, Ramsey NL *et al.* (1982). *Child and Family – Concepts in Nursing Practice.* McGraw-Hill Book Co., New York.

Tulman LJ (1985). Mothers and unrelated persons initial handling of newborn infants. *Nursing Research*; 34(4): 205–9.

Wagner P (1976). Testing the adaptation model in practice. *Nursing Outlook*; 24(11): 682–5.

Wolff P (1969). The natural history of crying, in Foss BM (ed), *Determinants of Infant Behaviour.* 4th edition, Methuen, London.

Wright S (1986). Developing and using a nursing model, in Kershaw B and Salvage J (eds), *Models for Nursing*, John Wiley, Chichester.

Further reading

Aggleton P and Chalmers H (1984). Models and theories – defining the terms. *Nursing Times*; 80(36): 24–8.

Fitzpatrick J and Whall A (1983) *Conceptual Models of Nursing* Brady Publishers, Maryland.

Müller DJ, Harris PJ and Whattley LA (1986). *Nursing Children, Psychology, Research and Practice.* Harper and Row, London.

Pearson A and Vaughan B (1986). *Nursing Models for Practice.* Heinemann, London.

Rambo BJ (1984). *Adaptation Nursing – Assessment and Intervention.* WB Saunders Co., Philadelphia.

Roy C (1971). Adaptation – a basis for nursing practice. *Nursing Outlook*; 19(4): 254–7.

4

Health visiting support of a family with a handicapped child based upon Orem's self-care model

Shirley Dean

The purpose of this chapter is to consider the use of Orem's model of nursing in offering health visiting support to a family where there is a baby with Down's syndrome. An example of a family situation is used as a basis for discussing the implications and potential effects of such a handicap and the nature of the health visiting intervention. Orem's model of nursing forms the theoretical framework for the care of the family; assessment and care plans are developed from the first home visit after the birth of the baby.

The family

Jenny Y is 26, and David Y is 30 years old. They first met the health visitor through an antenatal referral when Jenny became pregnant. Jenny attended antenatal classes at the health centre, and both parents were happily involved in the anticipation and preparation for the birth of their first child. Jenny's pregnancy was uneventful and ended with a normal vaginal delivery of a baby girl, Claire. The appearance of the baby led to a diagnosis of Down's syndrome, to be confirmed by chromosome test.

Both parents were together when told about Claire's condition and, although the news was given in an open and sympathetic way, they were understandably shocked and distressed, questioning why this should have happened when there was no family history of mental handicap or genetic abnormality. They found it hard to believe that their small newborn baby could have a problem of this kind.

In the period of crisis and anxiety following the birth of Claire, the health visitor's role included offering support and practical advice with the purpose of helping the family adjust to the situation. When considering the focus for health visiting intervention for the Y family some of the possible early effects of the birth of a baby with a handicap are reviewed.

The birth of a child with a handicap brings many consequences both immediate and long term, involving not only the infant but the parents and extended family as well. The effects will vary among individual families and this has implications for the professional worker offering support in the management of the child and the care of the family.

The parents' first reactions to the knowledge of having a child with a handicap may include conflicting feelings of shock, grief, anger and helplessness. Cunningham (1982) speaks of an instinctive reaction of protection towards the new baby combined with feelings of revulsion at the abnormality. Cunningham also indicates the extra stress that may affect first time parents who may feel a sense of 'reproductive inadequacy' in not producing a normal child.

There is evidence that the way in which the parents are told of the diagnosis is important. Byrne *et al.* (1988) found in the Manchester Down's syndrome cohort study the way in which the parents were told of the diagnosis of Down's syndrome during early visits to families had a significant effect on adaptation to the baby. Ideally, both parents are told together, with the baby present, and with time allowed for discussion. If the parents' perception is that the diagnosis was conveyed in an insensitive or unhelpful manner, this may adversely affect their view of the health professionals. This can be relevant for the establishment of a good professional relationship between health visitor and client, because as Allan (1987) points out, it is at this time that the health visitor becomes known to the family or consolidates an earlier contact.

The initial reactions are followed by a period of adjustment which Cunningham (1982) speaks of as lasting two to three months: he finds that a small number of parents never seem able to come to terms with the handicap, though most learn to live with their child and the handicap. For the parents of a first child extra problems may arise from not having had the experience of caring for a normal baby, and so they do not have confidence in distinguishing what is normal infant behaviour from that which results from Down's syndrome.

In addition to emotional support and the opportunity to express their feelings, families may require information about the nature of the handicapping condition and any developmental, medical or health problem likely to affect the care of their child[*]. In Down's syndrome, slow development in the early years, and learning difficulties are characteristic (Cunningham, 1982). Parents are encouraged to be involved in early intervention programmes to stimulate development. Berger and Cunningham (1983) emphasize the importance of parent–infant interaction in this, and the need for parents to understand that babies with Down's syndrome will smile later than non-handicapped children and will take longer in coping with and responding to stimulation.

Medical and health-related problems occur frequently with Down's syndrome. Aumonier and Cunningham (1984) studied a representative sample of infants with Down's syndrome aged 0–2 years and found medical problems of neonatal

jaundice (49 per cent of total sample); cardiac lesions (47 per cent); hearing impairment (45 per cent); and problems of vision (62 per cent); in addition, congenital abnormalities were found. Health related problems included fine, dry skin prone to soreness, irregular bowel action and poor peripheral circulation. Greater persistence was also needed to establish breast-feeding.

For the family there will be frequent contact with professional workers. The child's special health needs and educational needs will involve parents working with members of the health, education and social services at different times, depending on the child's stage of development. The parents' role as partners has been acknowledged since the Court report (DHSS, 1976). Christie (1986) regards the management of the child with a handicap as a dynamic process, with a team approach to assessment, treatment and long term care, including good communication and participation with parents.

Social consequences of handicap may affect the individual and the family, producing isolation and feelings of social stigma and difference. Some of this may result from labelling and stereotyping of the condition with negative impressions from the past, despite evidence that people with Down's syndrome may be able to live independent lives, as described by Laurent (1989), and that there are great variations among individuals. Booth (1985) argues that while people with Down's syndrome as a group may have varying degrees of physical impairment, and are relatively incompetent at some tasks when compared with the population as a whole, the extent to which they have a handicap depends on the way the individual is treated and the resources and opportunities made available to him or her.

Orem's model of self-care

Orem first described her model in 1959 and has subsequently developed and refined her original ideas. Central to Orem's model is the concept of self-care. Self-care is defined by Orem (1985) as 'the practice of activities that individuals initiate and perform on their own behalf in maintaining life, health and well-being' (p.84). Self-care

[*] Down's Syndrome Association, National Centre, Birmingham Polytechnic, 9 Westbourne Road, Edgbaston, Birmingham B15 5TN. Tel: (021) 454 3126. Also at 155 Mitcham Road, London SW17 9PG. Tel: (081) 682 4001.

activities are deliberate, learned behaviours, influenced by beliefs and culture, and are continuous throughout life. While adults normally undertake their own self-care, infants, the old or the ill may require complete or partial help with their self-care activities, and this is described as dependent self-care. Where individuals are unable to accomplish self-care activities or meet the self-care demands made on them, a self-care deficit is said to exist.

Orem (1985) identifies three types of self-care demands or requisites: these are universal, developmental and health deviation self-care demands. The universal self-care requisites are those common to all people and comprise the adequate intake of air, water and food, care associated with excretion, maintenance of a balance between activity with rest, balance between solitude and social interaction, the prevention of hazards to human life and functioning, and finally the promotion of human functioning and normality. Positive health and well-being are promoted when self-care or dependent care provided by a parent or a nurse is based on these requisites. Developmental self-care requisites are associated with human developmental stages such as infancy, and with conditions resulting from events in the human life cycle such as pregnancy. They also relate to the provision of care to prevent or mitigate problems that adversely affect development, which could include poor health, oppressive living conditions or difficulties in social adaptation. The third type of self-care requisites identified by Orem are health-deviation self-care requisites: these needs arise from disease, disability, or injury and can involve changes in human structure, physical functioning, and in behaviour and habits of daily living. Such changes can result in an individual becoming dependent on others either totally or to a lesser degree, and so moving in Orem's terms from being a self-care agent to a receiver of care, or a patient.

Nursing is seen by Orem (1985) as a helping system concerned with assisting people to maintain a balance between their self-care ability and the demands made on this ability. Where the self-care demand is greater than the individual's (or caregiver's) ability to meet it, nursing intervention will be needed. Orem describes three systems of nursing which are implemented according to individuals' capacities to care for themselves. Firstly, in the wholly compensatory system, the nurse will undertake actions for a patient unable to perform self-care, as in severe illness. In the second or partly compensatory system, both nurse and patient perform care measures that involve manipulative tasks and ambulation. The patient's physical abilities and psychological readiness and the knowledge and skills required will determine the relative responsibilities of nurse and patient. The third nursing system, the supportive–educative system, is particularly relevant to health promotion, and is used when the client is able and can learn to carry out self-care. The nurse's role may be supportive, educative, or consultative.

Five possible methods of helping may be used by the nurse. These involve acting for another person, guiding and directing, providing physical or psychological support, providing an environment that supports development, and teaching (Orem, 1985). The method of helping will reflect the nursing system employed. In the course of one illness a patient may range from being a dependent recipient of care, to performing activities in co-operation with a nurse, to being a learner developing knowledge and skills required for self-care.

In Orem's model of self-care, health is perceived as the 'state of wholeness or integrity of human beings' (Orem, 1985, p.173) and the physical, psychological, interpersonal and social aspects of health are seen as 'inseparable in the individual'.

The individual functions as an integrated whole, maintaining health through self-care activities. Nursing may be needed when individuals are unable to initiate or implement self-care for themselves. Investigative procedures determine whether a self-care deficit exists; an appropriate nursing system will be used to meet this. Evaluation of the nursing intervention will be based on whether the patient's ability for self-care improves, and whether the self-care deficit decreases.

The choice of Orem's model for health visiting practice

In choosing to work with a particular model of nursing, Aggleton and Chalmers (1986) suggest that it is necessary to consider whether 'the concept of the patient, the role of the nurse and the values with which the model works are in accordance with what [is held] to be true to good nursing practice today' (p.70).

In Orem's model the view of health that encompasses psychological, emotional and physical aspects, and the concern with integrated human functioning to achieve and maintain health, seem compatible with the underlying principles of health visiting practice. The principles of health visiting are based upon a belief in the value of health, and comprise the search for health needs, the stimulation of awareness of health needs, the influence on policies affecting health, and the facilitation of health-enhancing activities (Council for the Education and Training of Health Visitors – CETHV, 1977.)

The practice of health visiting 'consists of planned activities aimed at the promotion of health and the prevention of ill-health' (CETHV, 1977). The concept of self-care is relevant to health promotion, and applies to healthy individuals as well as the ill; and self-care continues throughout life. Cheetham (1988) demonstrates the capacity for self-care in a ten month old baby and Chavasse (1987) found a surprising degree of self-care in an elderly and dependent patient. Orr (1985) considers that the development of the self-care concept will 'result in educating the individual to maintain and improve the state of well-being' (p.91). The health visiting intervention with the Y family will involve a long-term health teaching and supportive role that falls within the supportive-educative nursing system described by Orem.

Orem sees the nurse's role as complementary to that of the patient in providing self-care. This is relevant for health visiting where the establishment of a relationship with clients is essential to professional practice. Orr (cited Health Visitors Association – HVA, 1987) speaks of health visitors being 'concerned not with doing things for clients' but 'involved in doing things with the client' (p.17). The relationship envisaged between the Y family and the health visitor is one of partnership, empowering the family to make decisions and take action to meet their own health needs.

The goal of Orem's model is to promote self-care in individuals and in those providing dependent care for children. This presents a positive perspective for a family with a child with Down's syndrome, recognizing and valuing Claire's potential for development, and her parents' role in caring for her and for themselves with professional support. The investigative procedures outlined in the model emphasize the careful calculation of self-care deficits so that health visitor interventions will be appropriate and sensitive to the family's needs (Figure 4.1).

Using the model as a framework for care

The assessment was made at the time of the first post-natal visit to the family when Claire was two weeks old, and was reviewed at each subsequent visit. Some information about the family was already known as Jenny had met the health visitor antenatally and had been attending parentcraft classes. Assessment of the self-care needs of all the family was organized with reference to Orem's universal self-care requisites (Figure 4.2). In addition, Claire's age and diagnosis of Down's syndrome required assessment of her health deviation and developmental requisites. Assessment was also made of Jenny's developmental self-care needs in view of her recent pregnancy.

The assessment procedures in this model are detailed and thorough requiring the collaboration of the health worker, client and family. The first step in the nursing process is 'the initial and continuing determination of why a person should be under nursing care' (Orem, 1985, p.224). It results in judgements about the client's state of health, and decisions about what is to be done. Information is sought in order to determine the client's self-care demand and whether the individual can meet this. If a self-care deficit is

Self-care requisites Universal	Self-care ability	Dependent self-care	Self-care deficit and reasons
Maintaining adequate intake of air.	Breathing normally though potentially susceptible to respiratory infection.	Parents provide care and understand aspects of safety in maintaining this.	Parents lack adequate information about potential problems and how to recognize signs of ill-health.
Maintaining adequate intake of food and water.	Slow to feed: rather weak sucking ability. Slow weight gain.	Breast-feeding, do not wake baby for feeds if asleep.	Claire is slow to feed. Jenny does not realize the need sometimes to wake her for feeds.
Care associated with elimination and hygiene.	Passing urine normally. Bowel action × 1–2 per day.	Jenny gives all care associated with hygiene, understands need for hygiene in relation to feeds and elimination. Uses disposable nappies.	Tendency to sore buttocks. Claire has fine delicate skin.
Maintain balance between activity and rest.	Rather sleepy baby.	Care provided by parents.	Lethargic baby.
Maintenance of balance between solitude and social interaction.	Requires total care.	Parents aware of need to provide stimulation. They talk to her, and cuddle her but are not confident.	Uncertainty about ability to meet baby's needs.
Prevention of hazards to human life and functioning and well-being.	Requires care.	Alert to physical hazards. Parents live in a warm, well-furnished house: maintain a safe environment.	None identified but may need guidance as Claire develops in relation to prevention of physical, social and emotional hazards.
Promotion of normality.	Requires care. May be slow to respond to stimulation.	Parents very anxious for Claire to achieve her full developmental capacity but uncertain as to how to do this.	Parents need more information and support from HV and other workers e.g. Child Development Unit, PHCT, Down's Syndrome Association.
Developmental Opportunity to develop.	Potential is present.	Parents anxious to do this, have some uncertainty and lack confidence.	Need for support and advice and profession intervention, eg. portage, physiotherapy.
Evaluation of development.	Requires care.	Parents have some knowledge of this and are aware of use of health services for child health surveillance.	Parents lack understanding of the process of development. Require anticipatory guidance. Claire will need regular assessment.
Protection against infection.	Has some capacity.	Aware of Claire's general need for care, and accept immunization programme.	Will require immunization.

Figure 4.1   Assessment of Claire

Self-care requisites	Self-care ability	Dependent self-care	Self-care deficit and reasons
Health deviation			
Physical functioning.	Has Down's Syndrome, slight heart murmur, hypotonic, and has very fine sensitive skin.	Able to provide care, and have good potential ability. Need specific guidance and support.	Need appropriate knowledge regarding handicapping condition, and how Claire is affected.
Developmental progress.	Has potential for development though will need appropriate stimulation specific to her condition. Development may be slow, and process of bonding gradual, possibility of defects of vision and hearing.	Well-motivated to give care, though may be too enthusiastic in promoting Claire's development, and have unrealistic expectations.	Need for advice in helping Claire to develop and to work in partnership with professionals. Need for regular assessment. Need to understand how development in a Down's syndrome child will be different from a normal infant.

Figure 4.1   Continued.

shown to be present, its nature and the reasons for it are investigated, an assessment is made as to the suitability of engaging in self-care, and the potential for future self-care. Orem is emphatic that decisions about the need for nursing care should be made in the context of an effective relationship between client, family and the nurse. In the case of the Y family, the relationship between the health visitor and the family was initiated before Claire's birth and developed continuously through subsequent contact. Jenny and David participated in the assessment of their health needs. On the first home visit, Jenny was explicit about wanting to help Claire reach her full potential, but also identified her own uncertainty as to how this could be done. The assessment demonstrated not only self-care deficits, but also the parents' considerable ability and motivation to carry out their own self-care and the dependent care of Claire.

Robertson (1988) points out that the health needs of handicapped children will be similar to those of other children except for special requirements relating to their handicap. The assessment of Claire helped Jenny and David to recognize that they were meeting her needs for loving care, warmth and nutrition and that they would work

with appropriate professionals in the event of special needs such as promoting Claire's development.

The goals for health care were identified jointly between the parents and the health visitor and a plan of care was formulated (Figures 4.3 and 4.4). A considerable number of self-care deficits were identified and health care plans addressed most of these; however some goals took priority. One of these was the promotion and maintenance of breast-feeding. Aumonier and Cunningham (1984) state that there are many infants with Down's syndrome who have early feeding problems possibly due to hypotonia, weak sucking reflexes and placidity, so that breast-feeding takes longer to establish than in normal babies. Another health goal that required early intervention was to develop Jenny and David's confidence in caring for Claire and allowing them to express their feelings.

Other health goals related to potential self-care deficits such as possible respiratory infection in Claire and post-natal depression in Jenny (Figures 4.3 and 4.4). These goals reflected the health visitor's role in preventing any deterioration in condition. Longer term health goals to be addressed included David's cessation of smoking.

Self-care requisites	Self-care ability	Self-care deficit	Reason for deficit
Universal Maintaining adequate intake of air.	Normal ability in breathing.	David smokes 10–15 cigarettes per day – aware of potential effects.	Reluctant to stop. David says he will give up smoking soon but not now.
Maintaining adequate intake of water and food.	Adequate nourishment.	None	
Care associated with elimination and hygiene.		None	
Balance between activity and rest.	David works long erratic hours as a sales representative. Jenny is feeling tired with care of new baby, not sleeping well.	David feels tired sometimes, and rather tense at the moment. Jenny is getting insufficient rest.	This deficit relates to the care of the new baby, and anxiety about her and trying to cope with the stresses of this.
Balance between solitude and social interaction.	Enjoy being together; also have local friends. Extended family (Jenny's parents) live nearby and visit. At the time of assessment were not feeling like meeting people though talking of doing so soon.	None identified now but potentially may become isolated if they withdraw from contact with other people because Claire's condition makes them feel different.	Potential deficit might develop.
Prevention of hazards.	Good home circumstances, with no obvious dangers. Other hazards relating to lifestyle not explored, but will be on later contacts.	None identified – may need anticipatory guidance.	
Promotion of normality.	Do not feel normal parents, though are enjoying looking after Claire.	Have not yet accepted or adjusted to Claire's condition. As yet have insufficient confidence and lack information as to the outcome of Claire's development.	Will need time to come to terms with Claire's Down's syndrome diagnosis, and work through feelings of distress and shock.

Figure 4.2   Assessment of Jenny and David

Self-care requisites	Self-care ability	Self-care deficit	Reason for deficit
	Still distressed by the diagnosis, and questioning Claire's management and future. Well motivated to giving care, and want to talk about this.		
Developmental (Jenny) relation to pregnancy and birth. Adjustment to new role.	Claire was a very much wanted baby. Jenny supported well by David, and extended family and friends. Has attended antenatal class whose members will form a post-natal group – these have been in touch.	Still in process of taking on new role, with extra stress as a result of Claire's handicap. Need for awareness of the possibility of post-natal depression.	Has not yet adjusted to new role which may take a considerable time. Will need continued support from family and friends, also from professional workers.
Maintaining breast-feeding.	Understands need for good nutrition, rest, and well supporting bra. Demand feeding.	Does not realize that it may be necessary to wake Claire to feed.	Claire has weak sucking reflex. Sleepy baby.
Post-natal care.	Post-natal examination arranged, and has contraceptive advice. Motivated to use, and has knowledge of services offered by health centres.	Aware of need to do pelvic floor exercises but inclined to forget.	Does not see that pelvic floor exercises are particularly important.

Figure 4.2   Continued.

While David recognized the need for this and had actually reduced his cigarette consumption, he did not feel able to stop smoking altogether at that time.

Assessment had shown that Jenny and David were well-motivated towards self-care and the plan of care was designed to meet their needs for support and help in caring for Claire and maintaining their own health. The health visiting intervention came within the supportive-educative system of nursing outlined by Orem (1985). It involved the health visitor making herself available to the family, by listening and giving Jenny and David time to express their feelings and talk about their concerns for Claire, and reinforcing their own ability to care for her. It also involved liaison with other workers in the multidisciplinary team concerned with the family.

Evaluation when using Orem's model of self-care would centre on whether the family have increased their ability in self-care, and whether

Health needs/deficit	Health goal	Plan/implementation	Review
Parents lack knowledge about potential problems and possibility of respiratory infection.	To increase knowledge. Jenny and David will recognize signs of illness.	Educative intervention (HV) to advise regarding early signs of illness. Regular developmental assessment.	Evaluation of parents increased knowledge – over long period of time.
Slow to feed.	To promote breast-feeding and good nutrition.	HV to discuss management of breast-feeding. HV to maintain centile chart. Jenny to breast-feed on demand, to wake Claire if necessary for 6 feeds per day. Long term: discussion of weaning.	Weekly review to assess progress and weight gain.
Tendency to have sore buttocks, chapped skin.	Action to prevent soreness of skin.	Frequent change of nappy, care in drying skin. Use of oil, cream.	Review progress at next visit.
Quiet, sleepy baby.	Opportunity for a variety of stimulation.	Jenny to give opportunity for interactive play. To have support from the Child Development Unit.	Review at each visit.
Parents uncertain about their own ability to meet Claire's needs.	Parents will feel able to look after Claire, and enjoy role of parents.	Educative supportive intervention by HV to encourage this. Jenny will contact HV whenever necessary.	Review at each visit for signs of developing confidence.
Protection against hazards.	Claire is not exposed to physical mental or social hazards. Immunization will be carried out. Parents will know reasons for this.	Anticipatory guidance regarding development and safety. Educate as to other hazards. Parents will have Claire immunized.	Attendance for immunization.

Figure 4.3   Care plan for Claire.

self-care deficits have been reduced. In the Y family one might look for signs of confidence in the management of care, for acceptance of Claire's handicap, and for Jenny and David to feel happy in their role as parents with less need for guidance and support. Claire, too, could show growing ability in self-care as she progresses developmentally. In a family with a handicapped child, achievement in self-care may be a slow process and evaluation will extend over a long period of time. Orem's model of self-care seems appropriate for health visiting practice in the community and offers a useful framework for working with a family where there is an infant with Down's syndrome. The central concept of self-care in which individuals are seen as carrying out actions to promote their health, the com-

Health needs/deficit	Health goal	Plan/implementation	Review
David smokes 10–15 cigarettes a day.	David will be a non-smoker	Long-term goal. No plan formed.	
Jenny is feeling very tired.	Jenny will not suffer from fatigue, will develop feeling of well-being	Jenny will rest during the day, and will accept offers of help from her mother. Take nutritious diet.	Review at next visit.
Potential isolation	To maintain and consolidate social contacts.	Will continue to see friends, and speak about Claire's handicap.	
	Jenny will adjust to new role of mother.	Jenny will join post-natal group.	
Coming to terms with Claire's handicap.	Parents will make be able to accept this emotionally.	HV will allow time for Jenny and David to talk about their feelings.	Evaluation continues over several months at least for signs of acceptance.
	Jenny and David will be knowledgeable about Down's syndrome.	Educative intervention and support for parents to understand syndrome.	
	Jenny and David will work with other professionals concerned with Claire and will feel supported.	HV will liaise with other workers who are or will be involved in decisions – programmes to stimulate Claire's development.	
	Parents will know about voluntary organizations.	Information given about Down's Syndrome Association.	Review whether Jenny and David will contact organization.

Figure 4.4   Care plan for Jenny and David.

prehensive view of health and the supportive-educative nursing system are compatible with health promotion and the health visitor's role compatible with a mainly well population.

Other models have been shown to have relevance to health visiting by Clarke (1986), Bach (1987) and Cowley (1988). Furthermore, Orem's model is not without potential difficulty in relation to the concept of self-care. Rosenbaum (1986) suggests that a model of self-care might be inappropriate in cultures which do not value self-care. While the goal

of self-care seems suitable for a family living in the Western world, an over-emphasis on self-care has the potential of leaving individuals to cope without adequate support.

The continuous nature of assessment in Orem's model is relevant for working with a family over a long period of time. The health visitor may have contact with a family for several years during which self-care ability may change and develop in both the adults and the children in the family.

The detailed investigative procedures in Orem's

model involve the client and lead to a good understanding of any self-care deficit and necessary nursing intervention. The baby who is handicapped needs to be treated as a normal baby as well as having special requirements. Using Orem's model helps to avoid the situation in which 'we may emphasize the handicap and fail to see the child beneath the handicap' (Aumonier and Cunningham, 1984, p.138).

Orem's model has much to contribute to health visiting practice. In using a model of self-care, the part played by the family is fully recognized and encouraged, leading to empowerment of clients to make informed choices as to their own health care. This model is also valuable for working with a family with a handicapped child; the potential for self-care can be demonstrated early and self-care ability encouraged, so that the family unit may be able to function to its greatest capacity.

References

Aggleton P and **Chalmers H** (1986). *Nursing Models and the Nursing Process*, Macmillan Education, London.

Allan E (1987). Down's syndrome and the health visitor. *Health Visitor*, 60(10): 335–8.

Aumonier M and **Cunningham C** (1984). Health and medical problems in infants with Down's syndrome. *Health Visitor*, 57(5): 137–40.

Bach S (1987). Evaluating the health visiting process using a model of nursing. *Health Visitor*, 60(9): 292–3.

Berger J and **Cunningham C** (1983). Early social interaction between infants with Down's syndrome and their parents. *Health Visitor*, 56(2): 58–60.

Booth T (1985). Labels and their consequences, in Lane D and Stratford B (eds) *Current Approaches to Down's Syndrome*. Holt, Rinehart and Winston, London.

Byrne E, Cunningham C and **Sloper P** (1988). *Families and their Children with Down's Syndrome: One Feature in Common*. Routledge, London.

Cheetham T (1988). Model care in the surgical ward. *Senior Nurse*, 8(4): 10–2.

Christie PN (1986). Management of the handicapped child. *Midwife Health Visitor and Community Nurse*, 22: 67–9.

Chavasse J (1987). A comparison of three models of nursing. *Nurse Education Today*, 7: 177–86.

Clark J (1986). A model of health visiting, in Kershaw B and Salvage J (eds) *Models for Nursing*, John Wiley, Chichester.

Council for the Education and Training of Health Visitors (1977). *An Investigation into the Principles of Health Visiting*. CETHV, London.

Cowley S (1988). In search of a model for health visiting. *Health Visitor*, 61(5): 149–51.

Cunningham C (1982). *Down's Syndrome: An Introduction for Parents*. Souvenir Press, London.

DHSS (1976). *Fit for the Future*. Report of the Committee on Child Health Services. Cmnd. 6684. Chairman: Professor SDM Court. HMSO, London.

Health Visitors' Association (1987). *Health Visiting and School Nursing Reviewed*. HVA, London.

Laurent C (1989). People with propects. News Focus. *Nursing Times*; 85(20): 16–7.

Orr J (1985). Assessing individual and family health needs, in Luker K and Orr J (eds) *Health Visiting*. Blackwell Scientific Publications, Oxford.

Orem D (1985). *Nursing: concepts of practice*, 3rd edn. McGraw–Hill, New York.

Robertson C (1988). *Health Visiting in Practice*. Churchill Livingstone, Edinburgh.

Rosenbaum J (1986). Comparison of two theorists on care: Orem and Leininger. *Journal of Advanced Nursing*, 11: 409–19.

5

Caring for a child undergoing a circumcision using Roper's model of nursing

Kathryn Jones and Alison While

Introduction

This chapter applies the nursing model of Roper *et al.* (1980) to the care of a six-year-old boy undergoing circumcision (removal of the foreskin) as a day patient. Day surgery is increasingly employed as health authorities seek to maximize their limited resources. The short-stay nature of the type of care makes it essential that nursing care is well planned to ensure that the children and their families received a good quality care.

Day surgery

In an attempt to maximize limited economic resources, alternatives to conventional hospital in-patient stays are an increasing feature of paediatric care. Indeed, value for money is emphasized in government publications (DHSS, 1989) and it has been suggested that the proportion of children undergoing day surgery may further increase. However, the advantages of day surgery also include the reduction of emotional trauma associated with hospital residence (Jackson, 1978; Campbell, 1987) and reduced incidence of hospital-acquired infections (Howell, 1974; Atwell and Gow, 1985). From an economic perspective, day surgery has the potential to permit a reduction in hospital bed provision (Atwell, 1974), a reduction in nurse labour costs through avoiding a 'unsocial hours' payments and the maximization of

parental caring abilities (Edwardson, 1983; Sainsbury *et al.*, 1986).

However, the very nature of day surgery means that children and their parents experience a more hurried process than in-patient peers (Sinclair and Whyte, 1987) and this lack of time in hospital is combined with parents being given additional responsibility for managing their child's recovery at home (Atwell and Gow, 1985). Sinclair and Whyte, (1987) have identified this lack of time as potentially reducing the preparation these children receive prior to surgery. Rodin (1983) has rightly asserted that parents are the most appropriate people to prepare children for hospital; however, the empirical evidence of Harris (1979), the Consumers' Association (1980) and Dobree (1989) suggests that parents lack the necessary information with which to carry out child preparation.

Day surgery usually demands that parents institute pre-operative fasting prior to hospital admission. Instructions relating to fastings should be included in the standard hospital letter and when carried out properly and combined with good hospital planning, children should be fasted ideally for six hours (Thomas, 1974). However, it appears that most children are fasted much longer (Thomas, 1974) which greatly increases the risk of hypoglycaemia (Welborn *et al.*, 1986) and furthermore, a prolonged fast is not only unpleasant for a child but will also delay the voiding of urine post-operatively and is therefore likely to be associated with an overnight stay. Such an outcome is undesirable from a variety of perspectives which include increased emotional trauma, family inconvenience, and inefficient use of hospital resources.

Not all surgical procedures lend themselves to day surgery (Royal College of Surgeons, 1985) and further Pineault *et al.* (1985) found that certain surgical procedures have inferior outcomes when carried out as day surgery. The most appropriate procedures involve relatively minor elective surgery necessitating only minimal general anaesthesia such as circumcision, hernia repair, and minor plastic surgery.

Circumcision

Since Gairdner (1949) questioned the validity of routine circumcision in the young boy, the procedure has become relatively rare and is now carried out mainly for religious or medical reasons. The most recent survey (Butler and Golding, 1986) suggests that about six per cent of boys are circumcised, with half of these operations being carried out during admission to hospital.

The main medical indications for circumcision are phimosis (a tight foreskin which is difficult to retract); paraphimosis (when the foreskin is retracted and cannot be drawn forward again) and balanitis (inflammation of the surface of the head of the penis). There is evidence, however, that appropriate care of the penis of a young child can greatly reduce the need for circumcision (Griffiths, 1984).

Outline of situation

Tom is a six-year-old boy who was admitted to hospital for day surgery. He required a circumcision due to recurrent balanitis. This is usually a straightforward operation but there is a risk of post-operative haemorrhage. For this reason good post-operative care is essential with appropriate advice for his parents prior to discharge, so that they will be able to manage his recovery successfully.

Tom had some experience of hospital before his admission. He is one of five children living with his parents on a large council estate in South London.

He remembers his mother giving birth to his younger brother Robin last year, Wendy his three-year-old sister having her broken arm set in the accident and emergency department and Jim, his nine-year-old brother, having his tonsils out. His school had been included in a hospital liaison visit to the children's wards earlier in the year and he had attended the out-patients' department.

He was, however, a little anxious about coming into hospital mainly because his mother would not be able to stay with him because of the other children (she was still breast-feeding Robin). His father works shifts and could not arrange time off. He was admitted to hospital at 8.30 am on Tuesday morning and his mother came with him as Mary, his eldest sister, was able to take the other children to school and nursery. His surgery was scheduled for late Tuesday morning and he was expected to be discharged on Tuesday evening.

Selection of a model, including rationale for choice

A model of nursing is a framework or guideline which attempts to organize and rationalize the nursing care given to an individual or group of patients. Roper's model of nursing is based upon a functional assessment of the activities of living (Roper *et al.*, 1980). Roper's model of living considers that a person's life is a continuum from conception to death during which his ability to look after himself may vary. Roper uses 12 activities of living (AL) to assess a person's ability to look after himself. These AL are: maintaining a safe environment; communicating; breathing; eating and drinking; eliminating; personal cleansing and dressing; controlling body temperature; mobilizing; working and playing; expressing sexuality; sleeping and dying. Roper states that a person's ability to be independent (or his position on a dependence continuum) will vary with both his age and circumstances e.g. whether he is handicapped or ill. The model assumes that even if a person is born handicapped he will not necessarily be totally dependent in all AL and that he may be able to progress along the dependence/independence continuum.

Roper's model of nursing looks at four areas of nursing:

- the patient's lifespan;
- his dependence/independence;
- circumstances affecting the patient;
- components of nursing.

Nursing is concerned with people throughout their lifespan and a person may be in need of health care at any point in his life. There are certain nursing specialists for specific areas of the lifespan, e.g. paediatric nursing, midwifery and geriatric nursing. The lifespan which is part of Roper's model of living and nursing reminds the nurse that her role is to care for her patients during all stages of life.

Roper's model of nursing further develops the continuum of dependence/independence introduced in the model of living. A child during the early years of life is relatively dependent upon others, whereas an adult is generally independent in all AL. As a patient this independence may alter, for example, an adult who has had an amputation may, at first, be totally dependent upon others to meet his mobility needs. However, with effective care and the provision of mobility aids he may progress to relative independence. During periods of illness or hospitalization, the nurse has a role in assessing a patient's level of independence with each AL, and appropriate nursing care is given depending upon circumstances. The patient may then travel along the dependence/independence continuum.

In Roper's model of living, circumstances suggested to affect a person's ability to perform AL are physical and mental handicap. During times of illness or hospitalization there are other influencing factors such as disturbed physiology, tissue changes, onset of illness, infection, accident or acquired mental and physical disability. It is important that a nurse basing her care upon Roper's model is able to understand why a person's usual routine has been altered so that she can provide appropriate care with short-term and long-term objectives.

Roper's model of nursing considers closely interrelated components of nursing. These are the AL-preventing, comforting and dependent components. The first describes all nursing activities carried out to meet a patient's needs with regard to AL. The preventing component seeks to protect a patient from harm caused by hospitals, for example, hospital acquired infection, stress induced ailments and complications arising from being in bed. The comforting component describes what lay-people see as the arts of nursing, such as positioning pillows to make a patient comfortable. The dependent component of nursing describes those duties a nurse carries out as a member of a multi-disciplinary hospital team, including drug administration, surgical dressings and passive limb movements.

In order to provide nursing care tailored to individual routines and habits, an assessment of the patient's usual routines and habits is made using the 12 AL as a framework, thereby ensuring that each aspect of his lifestyle has been considered.

Rationale for the use of Roper's model

Paediatric nursing has been developing as a speciality since the 1950s when the Platt Report was published (Ministry of Health, 1959). This report outlined the needs of children and their parents within health care and nursing and aroused sufficient public interest to inspire the inception of NAWCH (The National Association for the Welfare of Children in Hospital). Parents today are encouraged to be resident with their children in hospital (Jolly, 1988), and often carry out most of their children's care with help from nursing staff (Casey and Mobbs, 1988). Indeed there are some centres where nursing staff have an educative role only, teaching parents to care totally for their children (Sainsbury *et al.*, 1986). Roper's model of nursing lends itself well to the assessment of a child's independence in AL and the amount of assistance he needs from his main caregiver. The child and caregiver can be thought to travel together as a unit along the dependence/interdependence continuum. The model also permits the planning of nursing care to facilitate parents in their quest to continue their child's usual routine while in hospital.

It has been suggested that repeated hospitalization can affect a child's development and can in some cases lead to regression (Quinton and Rutter, 1976). Effective developmental assessment with each hospital visit is therefore useful as an aid to assessing a child's well-being. Roper's model of nursing can be used to assess a child's general development as each of the 12 AL can be influenced by physical, intellectual, emotional and social factors. By providing the opportunity for regular assessment, Roper's model is a valid choice for paediatric nursing.

Tom's expected hospital stay was eight hours. The aim of paediatric nursing is to alter a child's usual routines as little as possible during his stay in hospital. The child is thought to feel secure in his usual routines. Much of the 'hands-on' nursing care for a child undergoing circumcision will relate to the physical aspects of the surgery (preparing him for anaesthetic, carrying out post-operative observations for bleeding). Roper's model can act as a framework or checklist to ensure that all his physical needs are met and is therefore well-suited to children admitted for short-stay surgery. However, it still enables nursing care to be given appropriately according to the child's needs and those of his family by considering his emotional needs (e.g. communicating, working and playing). The preventing component of Roper's model is applicable when giving advice to parents prior to their taking their children home from hospital. This advice is very important for the well-being of both child and family and the Royal College of Surgeons (1985) recommends that both verbal and written advice should be given.

In summary, Roper's model of nursing was chosen to meet the needs of Tom and his family while he was in hospital because it was hoped that nursing care organized according to his usual routine would reduce his anxiety and that of his family. Roper's model provided a method of assessment and caregiving, while the preventing component of the model provided a medium for pre-discharge advice.

Assessment of problems

An assessment of Tom's needs whilst in hospital was made using Roper's activities of living (AL). His stage of development with regard to each activity was considered (see Figure 5.1).

1. Maintaining a safe environment
Tom was admitted for surgery to be carried out under general anaesthetic. At times during his admission he would be unconscious or semiconscious and would be unable to maintain his own safety. The environment to which he was being admitted was potentially unsafe.
Goals: For Tom to be adequately prepared for theatre.
For Tom's safety to be considered at all times whilst in hospital.

2. Communicating
On admission Tom was six years old. He was admitted to hospital for surgery but did not consider himself unwell. He had a limited knowledge of his body's organs and was interested in how his body worked. He remembered being unwell when he had had balanitis and had stayed home from school. His mother had told him that the operation would stop that happening again. He was unhappy that his mother may not be able to remain with him. His mother was unsure of the nature of his operation.
Needs: For Tom and his mother to understand the operation he was having.
For Tom's mother to be as anxiety-free as possible.

3. Breathing
Tom's general health was good on admission. Potentially post-operatively he may not have been able to maintain his respirations.
Needs: For Tom's breathing to be effective after his operation as seen by pink extremities and unlaboured chest movements.

4. Eating and drinking
Tom was a fussy eater used to eating snacks and sweets instead of proper meals. He had not eaten or drunk since going to bed on Monday evening. He

was told that once he came back to the ward after surgery he would be able to drink.

Needs: For Tom's normal eating habits to be altered as little as possible.
For his mother to understand the importance of a healthy diet for growth and development.

5. Eliminating

Tom's normal bowel habit was to pass a soft stool daily. He passed urine without pain.

Needs: For Tom's normal elimination pattern to continue whilst in hospital.

6. Personal cleansing and dressing

On admission Tom undressed himself so that the doctor could examine him. His mother said that he was able to wash himself if organized properly.

Needs: For Tom to be clean and in an operation gown by 10 am.

7. Controlling body temperature

Potentially Tom would not be able to control his own body temperature post-operatively.

Needs: For Tom's axillary temperature to be 36–37°C.

8. Mobilizing

Tom was noted to be an active child on admission. He ran happily and was able to skip and jump. Post-operatively he may have been less mobile due to pain.

Needs: For Tom to mobilize post-operatively with as little pain as possible.

9. Working and playing

Tom was from a large family and enjoyed other children's company. He liked playing with cars and planes and watching T.V.

Needs: For Tom to be allowed to play.
For suitable toys to be provided for his play.

10. Expressing sexuality

Tom was a little shy about his impending operation. His mother was worried about his reaction to his surgery and whether it would affect his sexuality.

Needs: For Tom's privacy to be considered.
For his mother's anxiety to be as minimal as possible.

11. Sleeping

Tom had not slept away from his family before coming into hospital. He normally slept in a room with his brother, Jim.

12. Dying

This was not an immediate problem. However there is a risk of mortality following circumcision due to bleeding post-operatively.

Needs: For Tom not to bleed following surgery.
For Tom to be observed regularly for early signs of bleeding.

Evaluation and critique

Time constraints of day surgery care are an important factor and in this context Roper's model is attractive. Firstly, the model is easily understood and its emphasis upon physiological and physical aspects of the individual ensures that the care focuses upon the critical aspects of day surgery care. However, the model also accommodates the social, cultural and psychological environment and chronological age in the assessment of the AL (Roper *et al.*, 1985).

The current philosophy of paediatrics is that hospital admission should disrupt normal routine as little as possible. Roper's model permits the identification of such routines and therefore encourages the planning of care to accommodate a child's normal routine, so potentially reducing the extent of psychological upset experienced by a child. However, while the model is well suited to a short stay in hospital with the identification of a child's normal routine and his ability to be independent in each of the 12 AL, the model does not address itself to child development over time. Furthermore, the limited facility for the assessment of psychosocial needs may render the model inappropriate for longer hospital admissions when psychological well-being is an important consider-

1. Problem 12/6/90	Aim of care	Nursing action	Evaluation
Tom is six years old and has been admitted to hospital. His mother is unable to remain with Tom due to other young children in his family.	For Tom to be as secure as possible whilst in hospital. For his normal routine to be altered as little as possible.	– Show Tom and his mother around the ward. – Introduce Tom and his mother to staff members. – Show Tom his allocated bed space and allow him to unpack his things. – Explain typical hospital day to Tom and his mother including visiting hours. – Complete appropriate nursing documentation in order that his normal daily routine is recorded (nursing assessment). – Assess how his normal routine will be affected by hospitalization and explain this to him and his mother. – Provide toys for him to play with suitable for his age and needs. – Ensure mother has a paediatric unit booklet and telephone number.	12/6/90 8.30 am Tom and his mother admitted to ward. Tom appears inquisitive but relaxed. Is most concerned about not having had breakfast and a drink. 12/6/90 9.45 a.m. Has drawn pictures of himself going to theatre.
2. 12/6/90 Tom has been admitted for circumcision on 12/6/90 at 10.45 am. He needs to be safely prepared for theatre.	For Tom to be safely prepared for his operation.	– Ensure Tom wears a nameband with his name, age, hospital number and ward on it. – Ensure that the doctor explains the operation to his mother and obtains consent. – Ensure that the anaesthetist examines Tom before theatre. – Ensure Tom is starved for 6 hours. – Be available to answer any questions his mother or Tom may have. – Record baseline observations, weight and height. – Tom to be in a clean operation gown by 10 am 12/6/90 (mum not able to help).	12/6/90 Pre-medication due at 10 am (papaveretum and hyoscine). 12/6/90 Pre-med given – did not like injection.

Figure 5.1 Plan of care for Tom.

Problem	Aim of care	Nursing action	Evaluation
		– Allow Tom to play through any fears with appropriate toys and the use of appropriate nursing skills.	
3. 12/6/90 Tom has returned from theatre having had a circumcision. He returned to the ward at 12.00.		– Nurse Tom on his side with one pillow until recovered from the anaesthetic. Observe and record respiration rate $\frac{1}{2}$ hourly for 2 hours and then 4 hourly. Assess effort of breathing with each observation. – Have oxygen and suction available.	12/6/90 12.00 – conscious but not alert (resp. .20) 12/6/90 15.00 – more awake maintaining own airway without difficulty. 12/6/90 18.00 – no longer a problem.
1) He may not be able to maintain his own airway.	For him to breathe effectively as seen by pink nail and no chest recession (Respirations per minute 18–25).		
2) Tom may bleed following his surgery. He has no wound dressing.	For him not to bleed. For any signs of bleeding to be observed promptly. (increased pulse rate and decreased blood pressure).	– Observe Tom's wound for signs of bleeding and record his pulse rate at the same times that his respirations are observed. – Report any changes to the nurse in charge. – Take blood pressure if pulse rate alters from his usual pulse rate (90 b.p.m.)	12/6/90 12.00 – no oozing (Pulse 92). 12/6/90 16.00 – no bleeding. 12/6/90 18.00 – wound clean and dry, no bleeding.
3) Tom may be unable to control his body temperature.	Axilla temperature at 36–37°C.	– Observe Tom for changes in temperature at least hourly. – Record axilla temperature at least two hourly. – Provide adequate clothing and bed linen.	12/6/90 12.00 – Temp. 36°C. 12/6/90 18.00 – Temp. 37°C, looks flushed.
4) Tom may be in pain.	For him to feel as little pain as possible.	– Observe Tom at least half hourly for signs of pain (raised pulse, increased restlessness). – Administer analgesia as prescribed safely (had papaveretum 10 mg in recovery at 11.30 am). – Use appropriate nursing skills and intervention to make him comfortable. – Mother is with Tom. – Provide all nursing care with attention to Tom's emotional needs.	12/6/90 18.00 paracetamol 375 mg given with effect. 12/6/90 Mother here for most of the day.
5) Tom may be frightened because of his operation.	For him not to be frightened	– Mother is with Tom. – Provide all nursing care with attention to Tom's emotional needs.	12/6/90 Mother here for most of the day.

Problem	Aim of care	Nursing action	Evaluation
6) Tom may vomit if he eats and drinks too soon after surgery. He may become dehydrated.	For Tom not to vomit. For Tom to remain hydrated as seen by moist mucous membranes.	– Allow Tom sips of water as soon as he is alert. – Gradually increase volume of drink as he tolerates it. – Resume normal eating habits once Tom has recovered from his general anaesthetic.	12/6/90 16.00 Has had a drink and not vomited. 12/6/90. 18.00. Ate a small portion of jelly and ice-cream.
7) Tom may not pass urine following surgery.	For him to pass urine by evening of surgery.	– Provide adequate analgesia as prescribed by doctors. – Take Tom to the W.C. when able to walk or offer a urinal.	12/6/90 17.00. Passed 200 mls of urine.
4. 12/6/90 Tom has been seen by the doctors who are happy for him to be discharged. His mother is able to take him home at 8.00 p.m. when her husband can collect them.	For Tom to be safely prepared for discharge. For Tom's mother to be aware of any complications which may occur.	– Talk with Tom's mother so that she understands any physical symptoms which may occur e.g. inability to pass urine, risk of bleeding. – Explain any behaviour changes which may occur due to Tom's stay in hospital, e.g. clinging behaviour. – Dispense medications to take home as prescribed. – Be available to answer any questions Tom and his mother may have. – Arrange out-patients follow up as ordered by doctors. – Provide hospital phone number in case of queries. – Explain appropriate wound care to Tom and his mother. – Provide advice sheet outlining ideal home-care.	12/6/90 20.00. Discharged home. TTO's paracetamol. OPD 6/52. Return for wound check 1.52.

Figure 5.1 Continued.

ation in the light of research findings (Quinton and Rutter, 1976).

The success of day surgery is dependent upon parents managing their child's recovery at home (Atwell and Gow, 1985). The preventing component of care in Roper's model enables advice to be given to parents in respect of home care and the management of complications. This advice should be both verbal and written (Royal College of Surgeons, 1985).

However, the preventing component is more closely related to information-giving regarding the prevention of harm or disease rather than education-giving. This shortcoming means that the practitioner must be careful to interpret their role to include education and facilitation in order to maximize the caring abilities of parents. Indeed, perhaps one of the failures of paediatric nursing has been the absence of full partnership with parents in the care of their children in hospital.

However, Roper's model was a sound choice for planning Tom's care. The framework highlighted essential problems of day-surgery children and permitted an acknowledgement of his developmental status. The pertinence of the model for longer-stay admissions is questioned in view of their increased psychosocial needs and the importance of facilitating continued developmental growth. The model also needs to be further developed to facilitate nursing care by parents and their education for that role.

References

Atwell JD (1974). *Paediatric day-case surgery in Southampton.* Unpublished paper presented at NAWCH Conference, 16 October.

Atwell JD and Gow MA (1985). Paediatric trained district nurse in the community: Expensive luxury or economic necessity? *British Medical Journal*; **291**: 227–9.

Butler NR and Golding J (eds) (1986). *From Birth to Five.* Pergamon, Oxford.

Campbell M (1987). Children with on-going health needs. *Nursing* 3rd Series; **23**: 871–5.

Casey A and Mobbs S (1988). Partnership in practice. *Nursing Times*; **2 Nov**: 67–8.

Consumers' Association (1980). *Children in Hospital.* Consumers' Association, London.

DHSS (1989). *Working for Patients.* HMSO, London.

Dobree L (1989). Pre-admission booklets for patients awaiting surgery. Occasional Paper. *Nursing Times*; **85**: 42–4.

Edwardson SR (1983). The choice between hospital and home care for terminally ill children. *Nursing Research*; **32**: 29–34.

Gairdner D (1949). The fate of the foreskin. *British Medical Journal*; **2**: 1433–7.

Griffiths DM (1984). The health visitor and the foreskin. *Health Visitor*; **57(9)**: 275.

Harris PJ (1979). *Children, their Parents and Hospital: Consumer Reactions to a Short Stay for Elective Surgery.* Unpublished Ph.D. thesis, University of Nottingham.

Howell M (1974). *Domiciliary care of children in Birmingham – its history and development.* Unpublished paper presented at NAWCH Conference 16 October.

Jackson RH (1978). Home care for children. *Journal of Maternal and Child Health*; **3(3)**: 96–100.

Jolly J (1988). Meeting the special needs of children in hospital. *Senior Nurse*; **8(4)**: 6–7.

Ministry of Health (1959). *The Welfare of Children in Hospital.* Report of Central Health Services Council. Chairman: Sir Harry Platt. HMSO, London.

Pineault R, Contandriopoulos A, Valois M *et al.* (1985). Randomised clinical trial of one-day surgery, patient satisfaction, clinical outcomes and costs. *Medical Care*; **23(2)**: 171–82.

Quinton D and Rutter M (1976). Early hospital admissions and later disturbances of behaviour: An attempted replication of Douglas's findings. *Developmental Medicine and Child Neurology*; **18**: 447–59.

Rodin J (1983). *Will This Hurt?* Royal College of Nursing, London.

Roper N, Logan W and Tierney AJ (1980). *The Elements of Nursing.* Churchill Livingstone, Edinburgh.

Roper N, Logan WW and Tierney AJ (1985). *Elements of Nursing.* 2nd edn. Churchill Livingstone, Edinburgh.

Royal College of Surgeons (1985). *Guidelines for Day Case Surgery.* Commission on the provision of surgical services. Royal College of Surgeons, London.

Sainsbury CPQ, Gray OP, Cleary J *et al.* (1986). Care by parents of the children in hospital. *Archives of Disease in Childhood*; **61**: 612–5.

Sinclair H and Whyte D (1987). Perspectives on community care in children. *Recent Advances in Nursing*; **16**: 1–15.

Thomas DKM (1974). Hypoglycaemia in children before operation: Its incidence and prevention. *British Journal of Anaesthesiology*; **46**: 66–8.

Welborn LG, McGill WA, Hannallah RS *et al.* (1986). Perioperative blood glucose concentrations in pediatric outpatients. *Anaesthesiology*; **65**: 543–7.

6

Caring for a child with asthma using Orem's self-care model

Mark Whiting

This chapter is based upon the care of a young child, David, who has asthma. The period from David's first birthday until his third birthday is the central focus of the chapter, and Orem's self-care theory provides the framework against which David's care is described.

Asthma

Asthma is the most common respiratory disease of childhood, affecting up to twelve per cent of the child population. In the first year of life, around one in every ten children show the recurrent symptoms of asthma (wheeze, cough and breathlessness), though the majority of these will not go on to develop 'classic' asthma (Park *et al.*, 1986, Warner *et al.*, 1989).

Asthma is a disease that is characterized by recurring paroxysmal attacks of (usually) reversible airway obstruction which presents as an audible expiratory wheeze, spasmodic cough (often worse at night) and breathlessness. The symptoms arise directly from the airway obstruction, which has three discrete components:

- constriction of smooth muscle in the walls of the bronchi and bronchioles as a result of increased parasympathetic activity;
- oedema of the bronchial/bronchiolar mucosa;
- over production of tenacious, viscid mucus from goblet cells, and serous and mucus glands in the bronchial/bronchiolar lining.

It is generally accepted that childhood asthma occurs by virtue of a type 1 allergic reaction, variously described as hyper-sensitivity, hyper-reactivity or hyper-irritability. Allergens (antigens) arriving in the lungs react with an immunoglobulin compound (IgE) on the surface of mast cells in the endothelial lining of the bronchi and bronchioles. This leads to mast cell degranulation, resulting in the release of vasoactive amines including histamine and SRS–A (slow reacting substance of anaphylaxis). The release of these amines has a direct effect upon the endothelial lining, resulting in both oedema and increased mucus secretion. Additionally, parasympathetic stimulation to the smooth muscle is increased, resulting in constriction of the airway. The combined effects of these reactions lead directly to the development of the symptoms of asthma described above.

The hypersensitivity reaction of asthma may arise from a whole range of trigger factors. These may generally be described as extrinsic or intrinsic. Extrinsic factors give rise directly to the antigen-antibody reaction described above and include inhaled substances such as animal fur, grass and tree pollens, the house dust mite (*Dermatophagoides pteronyssinus*), and material fibres. Extrinsic factors also include foodstuffs, particularly milk and other dairy products or cereals. Intrinsic factors do not invoke this antigen-antibody reaction, and asthmatic attacks are triggered by a variety of mechanisms. They include psychosomatic triggers such as anxiety, excitement or fear, as well as exercise, bacterial or viral infections of the upper or lower respiratory tracts, inhalation of irritants such as tobacco fumes, or changes in temperature of inhaled air.

Childhood asthma is closely related to eczema and hay fever. Both extrinsic and intrinsic trigger factors are thought to contribute to the triad of atopy (definition) that is formed by the three conditions. All three have a familial tendency and a family history of atopy is very common in the young child with asthma.

Children who suffer from asthma can be conveniently divided into three groups depending upon the severity and frequency of symptoms:

Mild Group: These children suffer occasional attacks which are usually preceded by upper respiratory tract infections; they are symptom free between attacks. During the period between attacks, the children's pulmonary function tests (PFTs) and growth are normal. Bronchoconstriction may occasionally be induced by exercise, but often resolves spontaneously.

Intermediate Group: This group of children suffer from severe recurrent episodes, but are generally symptom-free between attacks. The attacks are commonly induced by exercise or respiratory tract infections, though specific extrinsic factors may be implicated.

Severe Group: Although within this group the severity of attacks may themselves vary, the child is rarely symptom-free. Growth and development as well as PFTs are considerably affected, PFTs being abnormal at all times.

Regardless of the severity or frequency of symptoms, the successful management of the child with asthma involves a complicated array of therapeutic and educative strategies which, in turn, rely heavily upon the cooperation of both the child and his family in an agreed plan of management. The management plan may be usefully discussed using just two headings, drug treatment and education for prevention.

Drug treatment

A wide range of chemotherapeutic agents are employed in the management of acute childhood asthma. Although it is only possible to summarize briefly the role of drug therapy in this chapter, the value of an effective regimen should not be underestimated. A number of specific groups of drugs form the mainstays of treatment:

Bronchodilators, such as salbutamol and terbutaline have an adrenergic effect upon the β_2 receptors of smooth muscle in the bronchial wall. Other atropine-like bronchodilators such as ipratropium bromide have a similar effect. Each of these preparations may be given as oral preparations or may be inhaled.

Theophylline derivatives such as aminophylline or theophylline itself also have an adrenergic effect and act as bronchodilators. They are often used as additional therapy with salbutamol or terbutaline. In general they are given orally, but may cause gastric irritation and may not be tolerated in either syrup or capsule form.

Steroids have an anti-inflammatory effect upon the bronchial lining, inhibiting the release of vasoactive amines (histamine etc.). Historically, high dose oral steroid preparations were employed in the management of asthma, but undesirable systemic effects limited their use. The introduction of low-dose inhaled preparations such as beclomethasone dipropionate and betamethasone valerate in the 1970s, provided a mechanism for administration which has proved acceptable and effective while eliminating the side-effects that were associated with oral therapy. The principal role of inhaled steroids is in prophylaxis; oral steroids being mainly employed as an emergency treatment.

Other prophylactic agents. Sodium cromoglycate is a widely prescribed substance which is only available as an inhaled preparation. It acts by stabilizing the mast cells in the bronchial lining and preventing cellular degranulation. Ketotifen has similar effects to sodium cromoglycate and is available as an oral preparation, however its efficacy is not yet well established. Terfenidine has an anti-histamine effect and, since its introduction in liquid form, it has been increasingly used in the management of childhood asthma.

Effective drug treatment relies upon close compliance with the prescribed regime. It is of crucial importance that the child's family appreciates the necessity for continued administration of medicine, particularly of prophylactic drugs, even when the child is completely symptom-free.

Education for prevention

As noted above, the role of the family in the successful management of childhood asthma is crucial. Warner *et al.* (1989), in a multi-national consensus statement on the management of childhood asthma, advise that:

> 'The management of asthma should be an example of shared caring in which the child, the parent and the medical advisors act as a team in managing the asthma.'
>
> (p.1069)

Central to the ability of a family to contribute to this 'shared care' is the requirement that the family possess an adequate understanding of both the condition itself and all aspects of its management. The family's role has two distinct components. In the first instance, it involves those actions which are aimed at prevention of acute asthmatic attacks, and secondly, it relies upon the appropriate management of an attack which is already in progress.

Although, as mentioned earlier, prophylactic drug therapy can make a major contribution to successful prevention, the identification of possible trigger factors is arguably of even greater importance. Every child's experience of asthma is different from that of any other and, although a vast range of trigger factors have been implicated, the identification of the specific triggers for a particular child may prove problematic. The child's family needs to be made aware, at an early stage, of some of the potential triggers in order that they can exclude or possibly confirm their significance for their own child. Education by medical and nursing staff about both possible trigger factors and effective methods of dealing with them is essential. In some children skin testing may be usefully employed, but, as a rule, a sound medical/nursing history may prove more valuable in identifying specific trigger factors. The child and his family, who will provide the source for such a history, may

then be enlisted in both a concerted attempt to further identify factors and also to limit contact with these factors, whether they be of an extrinsic or intrinsic nature.

As an example, although in childhood asthma symptoms are often worse at night, regular damp dusting of bedrooms, replacement of feather pillows with synthetic foam, regular washing of sheets and elimination of pets from bedrooms may all contribute to a reduction in nocturnal symptoms.

It is crucial that the family is fully conversant with the child's drug prescription, and they must be aware of the role of each drug and its importance within the overall regime. It is only when the family is given this information that they can realistically be expected to follow what is often an extremely complex timetable of administration. The use of an 'asthma diary' over a period of several months may be of particular value in ensuring compliance. It must be anticipated that the problem of poor compliance is most likely to occur at times when the child is symptom-free. However, once again a well-kept diary can itself be a useful adjunct to therapy in that it can often be used to illustrate retrospectively the relationship between drug compliance and reduction in symptoms.

The role of nursing and medical staff whether in the children's ward, out-patient department or community setting is clearly central in providing the child and his family with the necessary knowledge to enable them to make an effective contribution to the management of the child's asthma. It must be acknowledged, however, that a relatively short contact time is often available for direct professional intervention in the clinical setting. This in itself is likely to restrict the amount of information that can be given and clearly reinforcement is of vital importance. Increasingly, this reinforcement take the form of activity pamphlets and reading books (see p. 61) which the child and family can browse through at home and which can be used as a reference source for information, or by contact with self-help groups.*

The establishment of an appropriate balance of hospital and community nursing and medical input

* Asthma Society and Friends of Asthma Research Council, 300 Upper Street, London N1 2XX. Tel: (071) 226 2260.

into the management of the child with asthma may itself present a number of problems, some of which will be highlighted later. In a chapter of this size, it is not feasible to explore all of the potential sources of advice, support and treatment which may be available to the family. It is, however, necessary to emphasize at this stage that tremendous local variations do exist in the respective contributions of a whole range of health care professionals to the care of the child with asthma and his family. This will include the contributions of ward and out-patient nursing staff, hospital medical staff, community nurses including community paediatric nurses, district nurses, health visitors and school nurses, the general practitioner and hospital- and community-based physiotherapists.

In the section that follows, a number of aspects of the role of both formal health care agencies and of the family itself will be explored within a detailed account of the Orem self-care model, which the author believes provides a useful framework for discussion of the management of childhood asthma.

The Orem self-care theory

Of all the models and theories which have emerged from the efforts of nurses to provide a theoretical framework upon which to base their practice, the self-care theory of Dorothea Orem (1959, 1971, 1985) perhaps best lends itself to the care of the child with asthma. Within this section, the self-care model will be introduced and described in some detail. Following this, its specific application to the care of the child with asthma will be explored.

Riehl and Roy (1980) describe theory as 'a scientifically accepted principle which governs good practice or is proposed to explain observed fact'. This definition provides a useful starting point for discussing Orem's self-care theory. Although self-care cannot be described as a 'scientifically accepted principle', and is in fact based upon a number of assumptions which Orem herself has failed to explore in any detail (e.g. it is assumed throughout Orem's work that man's rationality causes him to take definite, decisive actions within the limits of his own abilities to maintain or restore

his health), the self-care notion is one that many nurses have been able to identify with and has allowed the theory to be applied in a wide range of clinical settings.

The theory was first presented by Orem in 1959. Self-care is defined as 'the production of actions directed to the self or environment in order to regulate one's functioning in the interest of one's life'. Orem suggests that an individual has self-care requisites (or self-care needs/demands) and that he is equipped with self-care abilities to help him manage his requisites. Orem further suggests that the ability of an individual to engage in self-care is conditioned by age, developmental stage, health status, life experience, socio-cultural orientation and availability of resources.

Orem identifies three types of self-care requisites:

Universal self-care requisites represent those human activities which are responsible for day-to-day maintenance and functioning. This particular concept aligns well with what are described elsewhere as 'activities of living' (Roper *et al.*, 1980) or 'activities of daily living' (Henderson, 1964).

Developmental self-care requisites were initially considered by Orem (1959) as falling within the category of 'universal self-care requirements' (later referred to as requisites), but subsequently Orem (1971) developed this particular sub-concept in its own right, and describes it as those requisites which are 'particularized for human development' (to include those requisites which arise out of the developmental immaturity of a young child) or are 'new requisites derived from a condition (such as pregnancy) or an event (e.g. loss of a spouse or parent)'.

The third area is that of *health deviation* self-care requisites, which arise only when health is threatened or compromised. This relates to those requisites arising directly or indirectly from any deviation from full health.

At a time of good health the individual is in a state of equilibrium in which self-care demand is constantly being satisfied by normal self-care abilities. Clearly, in respect of the young child whose self-care abilities are somewhat immature, the overall balance of self-care requisites is tilted toward developmental self-care requisites and in this regard, the role of the family, and the child's parents in particular, is crucial.

When an individual's health is compromised a self-care deficit may result. Orem suggests that an individual is equipped with reserve self-care abilities which will on occasion allow a return to the state of equilibrium without compromising the individual's general self-care status. The individual who suffers an imbalance in his self-care equilibrium is equipped with compensatory mechanisms which may allow for whole or partial compensation, and this may in turn result in recovery of the resting self-care status. In a child these compensatory mechanisms are rather limited and the ability of the child to restore a resting equilibrium relies heavily upon actions taken by his family rather than those that he might take himself. The relationships between self-care, self-care requisites, self-care abilities and self-care deficits are illustrated in Figure 6.1.

It is only when a person is unable to re-establish equilibrium through self-care and reserve self-care activities that additional intervention is required. In these circumstances intervention may be provided by another individual, and to describe such an individual Orem uses the term dependent-care agent. This term pertains to any agency that assists the individual in making up a shortfall in his/her self-care abilities. Re-establishment of equilibrium is achieved by partial compensation if the individual is able to contribute to health recovery or by whole compensation if unable to do so e.g. in the very young child. With regard to the care of a young child, the role of dependent-care agent is taken on in the first instance by his family and subsequently by those members of the health care team who are used as a source of advice, support and practical help.

The role of the dependent-care agent is described by Orem as supportive-educative. Although this description is almost self-explanatory, it gives some indication of the complexity of the nursing role in respect of the care of the child. Orem (1985) herself, acknowledges this:

'The nurse's dual relationship to child and to parents makes the nurse role complex and requi-

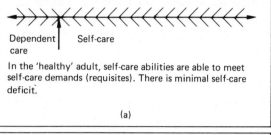

In the 'healthy' adult, self-care abilities are able to meet self-care demands (requisites). There is minimal self-care deficit.

(a)

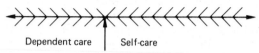

In the 'healthy' child self-care abilities are improving constantly, however developmental self-care deficits require parental/family intervention as a dependent care agent in order to maintain an equilibrium.

(b)

In the child with asthma, self-care abilities are compromised because a health deviation deficit is present. Parental family intervention (as well as nursing intervention) is required to restore the equilibrium.

(c)

Figure 6.1 The relationship between self-care and dependent care in the healthy adult and child, and in the child with asthma.

res that techniques of assisting be adapted to the needs of the child and the needs of the parent'.
(p.260)

Orem (1985) goes on to acknowledge that the developmental immaturity of the growing child influences the roles taken on by both nurses themselves and other dependent care agents (for example, the child's family).

'Nursing in situations where the patient is young may involve direct care of the patient by the nurse and assistance to parents or guardians in learning to give the continuous care needed by the child.'

(p.260)

Orem's theory is a very general theory of nursing, and has been applied across a wide range of patient/client groups. The inherent simplicity of the lynchpin concept of self-care has facilitated its widespread acceptance. However, in 1959, when the theory was first introduced, the concept of developmental self-care requisites was poorly defined and inadequately explained. This clearly restricted the possible application of the theory to the nursing care of children. By 1971, Orem further developed the theory and identified developmental self-care requisites as a separate concept. This has enabled the theory to be applied far more readily to child care.

Self-care and the child with asthma

As noted earlier, Orem describes three elements of the nursing role in meeting patients' self care requisites. These are wholly compensatory, partly compensatory and supportive-educative roles.

In respect of the care of a child with asthma, the predominant roles taken on by nursing staff are likely to be partly compensatory and supportive-educative. Only under extreme circumstances will the nurse be required to fulfil a wholly compensatory role (e.g. in providing care for a child with a severe acute asthmatic atack or in *status asthmaticus*). The role played by family members in the care of a child is primarily that of partial compensation, though, particularly in respect of the older child, a supportive-educative role is vital. The various roles of the nurse and family as dependent care agents are illustrated in Figure 6.2.

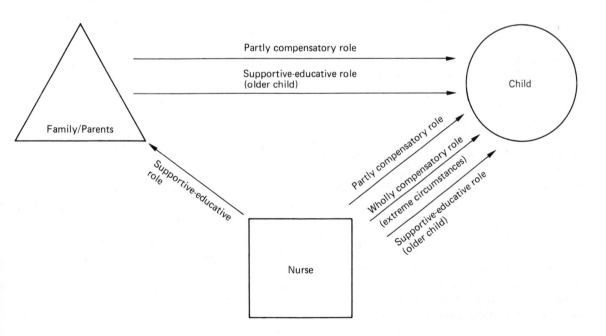

Figure 6.2   The roles of the nurse and parents/family in the care of a child with asthma.

The Orem self-care theory lends itself well to the care of the child with asthma, focusing as it does on:

- Practical care (when the nurse, as the dependent care agent, fulfils a partly/wholly compensatory role).
- Facilitating the re-establishment of self-care (when the nurse fulfils a supportive-educative role).

During an acute asthmatic attack, the role of the dependent care agent (whether that be a family member, nurse or other health professional) involves partially compensating for the health care deficit which arises out of the embarrassment to normal respiratory function. This role is primarily associated with the in-hospital care of the child. In the remainder of this chapter, however, the supportive-educative role will provide the principal focus for the plan of care and will be discussed in some depth. This role is fulfilled primarily by the nurse or other health professional. Such a role is vital in both maintaining the self-care equilibrium and in facilitating the family's own role as dependent care agents. As discussed earlier in the chapter, the need for the child's family to be equipped with appropriate information about the condition is vital if they are to take on such a role.

David

In this section, David, a young boy with asthma will provide an illustrative example of the application of the self-care theory. The period from David's first to third birthdays will be discussed. This will allow the identification of developmental self-care deficits arising as a result of David's age as well as specific health care deficits related to his asthma.

David is the second child of Susan and Danny M. His sister Yvonne is two years older, and the family live in a two bedroom, first floor council flat in north east London. Susan had mild hay fever for several years in her teens. Yvonne has mild eczema of her hands and elbows. Both Susan and Danny smoke approximately ten cigarettes per day. The family has two pet dogs and a cat.

David first developed respiratory symptoms at around nine months of age when, following a mild upper respiratory tract infection, he continued to cough, particularly at night, for two or three weeks. On the day following his first birthday, his mother brought him to the accident and emergency department of the local district general hospital with a two-day history of a runny nose and cold, for which the family general practitioner had prescribed amoxycillin. His runny nose and pyrexia was now accompanied by an audible expiratory wheeze and paroxysmal cough. David was given a single dose of nebulised salbutamol in the accident and emergency department and was admitted to hospital for overnight observation, accompanied by his mother. By the following morning he was completely wheeze-free, and, although his runny nose and occasional cough persisted, he was now apyrexial. No out-patient follow-up was considered necessary.

One month later, David was brought to the accident and emergency department by his parents. Once again he had symptoms of an upper respiratory tract infection. His runny nose had first been apparent that morning, and by early evening an expiratory wheeze had developed. David would not take any solid food, because every time he tried to swallow he started to cough. The family's general practitioner had visited him at home during the day and had suggested to Susan that he might be developing asthma and had prescribed amoxycillin and salbutamol syrup. David was admitted to hospital and was given aminophylline and hydrocortisone via an intravenous infusion. He was prescribed regular terbutaline nebulisers. Over the next thirty-six hours his symptoms showed a slow but steady improvement, the intravenous infusion was discontinued and prior to discharge David's mother was given a two-week supply of oral theophylline and terbutaline syrup as well as reducing doses of oral prednisolone. The importance of taking the medicines regularly was stressed to David's mother, though no additional details about the medicines were given at this stage. An out-patient appointment was made for one month after discharge, and the paediatric consultant explained to Susan that it was possible that David might have asthma.

Following discharge David remained symptom-free. His parents did not present him for his out-patient appointment, nor did he attend a subsequent appointment booked one month later.

Two weeks after this second failed appointment, Susan and Danny brought David to the accident and emergency department with an upper respiratory tract infection and symptoms of an acute asthmatic attack. Susan brought with her the almost-full bottles of theophylline and salbutamol as well as three unused prednisolone tablets. A blood sample taken for serum theophylline level showed a level of less than $1\mu g/ml$ (normal range 10 to 20 $\mu g/ml$). David's condition showed minimal improvement when given nebulised salbutamol in the accident and emergency department and so he was admitted, accompanied by Susan, to the children's ward. Overnight his condition showed little improvement despite regular nebulised terbutaline, and therefore an intravenous infusion of aminophylline was commenced.

When seen on the consultant ward round the following afternoon David's condition was much improved. He was referred to the community paediatric nursing team which was based upon the children's ward. The nursing team was asked to become involved in the management of David's asthma. A member of the community paediatric nursing team was present at the ward round, and so a formal written referral was unnecessary. The team member read through David's medical notes and ward nursing history/nursing care plan and the team then introduced themselves to David and his mother and gathered further details in order to produce a composite nursing history. A care plan was then drawn up using the Orem self-care theory as a basis for the identification of self-care deficits (nursing needs) and nursing interventions appropriate to those needs. This care plan is reproduced in detail in Figure 6.3 and sets out the focus of care provided to David and his family during the early months of contact.

The care plan is primarily concerned with nursing interventions related to the prevention of acute asthmatic attacks, but also considers some of the measures which the family might take during the early stages of such an attack. The care plan does not contain any reference to nursing interventions associated with any of David's in-hospital care following admission. In respect of the nursing interventions identified within the care plan, the nurse primarily fulfils a supportive-educative role, acting as the dependent care agent to the child and family.

On the ward round the paediatrician had re-inforced his earlier comments regarding the possibility that David was suffering from asthma. Prior to David's discharge from hospital, the community paediatric nurse met with Susan on two occasions. On the first occasion, the nurse added further details to the nursing history taken previously. Susan's understanding of the term 'asthma' was discussed and the community paediatric nurse explained briefly that many children suffered from asthma and that it was a condition for which a wide range of treatments and therapies were available. On the second occasion, Susan was supplied with a copy of the booklet *Your child and asthma*. The importance of taking regular medication was stressed to her and details of the medication regime were explained to both Susan and Danny. The nurse arranged to visit at home seven days after discharge. A two week supply of oral terbutaline syrup and oral theophylline syrup was given to Susan, together with an out-patient appointment four weeks later.

The community paediatric nurse visited at home the following week and further details were added to the nursing history. David had been symptom-free since discharge and Susan questioned the need to continue with his medication. The nurse stressed the necessity for strict compliance and Susan admitted that she had stopped giving David his theophylline because 'it makes him sick'. An attempt to give David his theophylline during this visit proved unsuccessful because David spat it out and started to retch.

Susan asked the nurse why David suffered from asthma. A lengthy explanation was given, including details of possible trigger factors. The possibility that cigarette smoke might be implicated was suggested and Susan was advised that she and Danny should try to avoid smoking at times when David was in the same room. Animal fur was identified as a further possible trigger factor. Susan asked whether the significance of possible trigger factors

Self-care deficit	Goal	Dependent care agent	Role of dependent care agent	Actions of dependent care agent
Developmental self-care deficits arising from David's 'normal' developmental immaturity.	To maintain a suitable environment for David so that he grows and develops within normal parameters.	David's parents (Danny and Susan).	Role comprises supportive-educative and partly compensatory elements.	Orem (1985) identifies eight universal self-care requisites: (i) The maintenance of sufficient intake of air. (ii) The maintenance of sufficient intake of water. (iii) The maintenance of sufficient intake of food. e.g. provision of well balanced diet. (iv) The provision of care associated with elimination processes and excrements. (v) The maintenance of a balance between activity and rest. e.g. provision of a 12 hour night sleep. (vi) The maintenance of a balance between solitude and social interaction. (vii) The prevention of hazards to human life, human functions and human well being. e.g. anticipation of childhood accident precursors, (viii) The promotion of human functioning and development within social groups in accord with human potential, known human limitations and the human desire to be normal.
Health – deviation self-care deficit to David as a result of limitation in respiratory function.	To maintain adequate respiratory function so that David has no episodes of respiratory insufficiency.	Community paediatric nurse and David's parents	Partly compensatory.	Observation and assessment of respiratory function. Provision of a suitable 'healthy' environment in which appropriate care can be given. Administration of prescribed medication. (i) in response to observed symptoms.

Figure 6.3   Care Plan.

Self-care deficit	Goal	Dependent care agent	Role of dependent care agent	Actions of dependent care agent
				(ii) in order to reduce the likelihood of symptoms occurrence (prophylaxis). Other strategies aimed at prevention of symptom occurrence, including (i) identification of potential trigger factors (ii) elimination of potential trigger factors, by, for instance damp dusting, no smoking instruction to guests at home, avoiding exposure to children with overt coryzal symptoms. Keeping pets out of David's bedroom.
Danny and Susan's developmental self-care deficit arising from their lack of knowledge in relation to David's health deviation, self-care deficit (see above).	To acquire new knowledge and skills in order to be able to take a lead role in the management of David's asthma.	Community paediatric nurse.	Supportive – educative.	Observe and assess present level of parental knowledge. Assess and determine parental capacity for learning and willingness/ ability to take on role. Identify specific areas of 'new knowledge' which parents will require. Identify specific learning strategies which can be employed, for example, demonstration of nebuliser, use of asthma diary, activity pamphlets and reading books, involvement of family in identification of possible trigger factors. Operate teaching plan based upon identified learning needs and parental capacity for acquisition of new knowledge and skills. Evaluate effectiveness of teaching strategies by monitoring parental performance and evaluating parental understanding of all necessary aspects of the managment and care of David's asthma.

Figure 6.3 Continued.

could be proven, and mentioned that the family's general practitioner had talked about the possibility of skin testing. It was explained that this might be useful in the future, but that the most important action was for Danny and Susan to try and identify things which they felt might have triggered David's asthma. At this time, the only possible trigger which could be identified was 'coughs and colds' which had preceded each of David's previous acute attacks. In view of Susan's interest in trying to identify possible trigger factors, a copy of the booklet *Asthma: The Detective's Story* was given to her.

Susan was advised to collect repeat prescriptions for theophylline and terbutaline from her general practitioner, and the necessity to attend the out-patient appointment was stressed.

Susan and Danny brought David to the paediatric asthma clinic three weeks later. Although he did not have any symptoms of an upper respiratory tract infection, a faint expiratory wheeze could be heard in all areas of his chest. Susan reported that she had not been giving the theophylline syrup because it caused David to vomit. Slo-phylline capsules were prescribed as an alternative to the theophylline syrup and it was suggested that Susan empty the contents of the capsule onto a spoon and mix with yoghurt, honey or jam. Susan reported that when she had visited the family general practitioner for a repeat prescription of David's medicines, it had been suggested to her again that David might have a skin test at the hospital. The paediatric consultant explained that he did not wish to skin test David at this time. Susan was given an 'asthma diary card' to complete in which she would be required to record details of both David's symptoms and his medication regime. An out-patient appointment was made for David to be seen in two months.

The community paediatric nurse, who was in attendance at the asthma clinic, arranged to visit the family at home the following week in order to assess David's progress.

When the nurse visited, although Susan had not completed the diary card very well, it was clear that David had not been given the Slo-phylline. Susan stated that she thought that David was well in himself and that the tertbutaline therapy was suf-

ficient. The nurse explained that the two medicines were different and that their actions were complementary to each other. The nurse stressed that the Slo-phylline would be particularly helpful in eliminating nocturnal symptoms, and demonstrated to Susan and Danny how to break open the capsules and mix the contents with yoghurt. David, who by this time seemed to be getting used to the nurse's visits, happily took the yoghurt and Slo-phylline from the spoon. Susan agreed that she would give the medication as prescribed. Susan and Danny were asked if they had been able to identify and possible trigger factors. Danny suggested that following a recent visit to the house of a friend who had been decorating, David had had a poor night with several episodes of coughing. The nurse agreed that this was quite a likely contributory factor and advised that Danny and Susan should continue to be vigilant. The nurse stressed the need to complete the asthma diary, if possible, and arranged to see the family at the next out-patient appointment six weeks later but made the offer that Susan or Danny could telephone the community paediatric nursing office if any problems arose in the meantime.

Three weeks later Danny was admitted to hospital with an acute asthmatic attack, despite the fact that Susan reported that she had given both the terbutaline and Slo-phylline exactly as prescribed. David made a rapid recovery. Susan suggested that even though David had a mild cold, his symptoms might have been made worse because his bedroom had been damp, and Danny had been re-wall-papering. Although the medical staff agreed that this was possible, it was decided that David should be given a home nebuliser. The community paediatric nurse arranged to deliver the nebuliser to the family home the following morning.

David was prescribed sodium cromoglycate nebuliser solution three times per day as prophylaxis, to be given in addition to the oral terbutaline syrup and Slo-phylline capsules. The nurse delivered two weeks' supply of all three medications together with a portable nebuliser, masks and tubing. The nurse demonstrated to Susan how to prepare the nebuliser solution for administration and explained to her how to care for the machine.

Although David had received several nebulisers at the hospital, he was somewhat uncooperative when sat on his mother's knee at home. He attempted repeatedly to remove the nebuliser mask and began to cry. The nurse advised Susan that, because it was expected that David would require nebuliser therapy for several months, it was important to establish a routine in which David would sit happily and breathe normally during administration. The nurse recommended to Susan that she give the nebulisers at well-spaced intervals during the day and that she try to give them at times when she could easily give up some of her own time to sit with David. It was further recommended that suitable distractions such as toys and reading books be used when possible.

The nurse explained to Susan that sodium cromoglycate was a preventative medicine which in nebulised form was particularly effective and increasingly being used in children of David's age. The importance of good compliance with the total medication regime was stressed and the importance of obtaining regular supplies from the family's general practitioner was emphasized. The asthma diary card, which had been completed during the previous month (even when David was in hospital), was amended to include the additional medication. The nurse arranged to visit the following week.

At the next visit Danny was at home alone with David. He demonstrated a fair understanding of David's medication regime but asked that the nurse explain the use of the nebuliser and the role of sodium cromoglycate in the overall regime. Danny questioned the fact that David was now receiving so many medicines and wondered how long this would be necessary. It was explained that although it was not possible to reduce the medication at this time, the regime would be reviewed every time David was seen by the hospital medical staff. Danny said that he would bring David to clinic with Susan for the next appointment.

At the next appointment, the family was seen jointly by the paediatric consultant and community paediatric nurse. David was very well, with no audible wheeze. He had been symptom-free since the nebulised sodium cromoglycate had been commenced, and both Danny and Susan felt happy with the progress that he was making. The asthma diary card had been completed, and indicated that the medication regime had been adhered to well. It was decided to discontinue the diary, but Susan suggested that she would continue to keep a diary of her own. The nurse arranged to visit the family six weeks later and an appointment was made to see David in the paediatric asthma clinic as an out-patient three months later. The paediatric consultant and nurse agreed that if David remained well his oral terbutaline syrup should be given only when considered necessary.

During the next twelve months David made very satisfactory progress. He was admitted to hospital on two occasions as a result of acute asthmatic attacks. Each admission was of three days duration and David required intravenous aminophylline and hydrocortisone followed by reducing doses of prednisolone on each occasion. Throughout this year David attended the paediatric asthma out-patient department regularly and he was seen at approximately three monthly intervals by the community paediatric nurse. Serum theophylline levels, which were checked each six months, were within the therapeutic range. Danny and Susan demonstrated a very good understanding of all aspects of David's management and showed an avid interest in acquiring information that might assist with David's care. David's medication regime remained unchanged throughout the year with the exception of those occasions during which he was admitted to hospital.

At two and a half years of age, David was admitted to hospital via the accident and emergency department with an acute asthmatic attack, accompanied by his mother and his sister, Yvonne. Danny had recently changed his job and was working away from home at the time. David had not slept very well during the first week that his father was away from home. Throughout the second week he was very fretful and was admitted to hospital with a pronounced expiratory wheeze on the Wednesday evening. Although David made quite a rapid recovery he remained very wary and fretful. On previous admissions he had been described as 'playful', 'adventurous' and 'happy'. Susan suggested that he was 'missing his dad'. The community paediatric nurse, who had been very involved with the family, commented to Susan that an element of psychological stress in a susceptible child like David, could make the likelihood of an acute attack all the more likely. David went home on Friday.

He was brought back to the accident and emergency department the following Tuesday evening where he was given a salbutamol nebuliser and then went home. The community paediatric nurse visited the next day and Susan explained that David had been upset every evening since his father had taken up his new job, and that he had become wheezy and breathless almost every evening. The nurse suggested that Susan recommence giving David his terbutaline syrup each evening, one to two hours before bed time during the week to see if his symptoms diminished. The nurse suggested further that Susan might spend time reassuring David that his father would soon be home. Susan asked the nurse to explain how David's asthma could possibly be made worse as a result of his upset. The nurse explained that stress often contributed to childhood asthma, and that anything which helped to reduce that stress might help to alleviate David's symptoms, and further advised Susan that she might spend time with David each evening while his father was working away from home, comforting, reassuring and perhaps distracting him. The nurse arranged to visit again two days later.

At the next visit, Susan reported that David had been given terbutaline each evening, that his nocturnal symptoms had diminished and that, although he was still quite fretful in the evenings, his sleep had been relatively undisturbed. The nurse arranged to see the family in the paediatric asthma clinic two weeks later, but suggested that Susan might telephone to arrange an additional home visit if David's symptoms recurred.

At the clinic Susan reported that David had been symptom-free since last seen, and observed that he had slept well during the night even when his terbutaline syrup had been omitted (by mistake). It was suggested that she might, therefore, discontinue the regular terbutaline, but re-introduce it if necessary. A further appointment was made for David to be seen in six months time.

David was visited at home two days before his third birthday. Susan described him as a 'normal lad'. She observed that occasional symptoms usually resolved without recourse to additional medication, but that regular early administration of terbutaline syrup was effective. Although there had been a time when she thought he would 'never get better' she now felt that his asthma was a 'minor problem' in which she was able to play a very active role.

Evaluation of the self-care model in childhood asthma

Philosophies pertaining to the care of sick children have moved inexorably towards the involvement of parents in that care (Cleary *et al.*, 1986; Casey, 1988). The need for that involvement to be based upon the informed participation of parents in a planned programme of care is central to the self-care ethos, and the above case study demonstrates how vital such participation can be. Many medical conditions give rise to chronic health deviation deficits in children (such as diabetes mellitus, cystic fibrosis, sickle cell disease, and congenital heart disease). The study of the care of a child with asthma described here, provides a very valuable illustration of the potential of the self-care model for identifying the problems and needs of such children and their families. The underlying principles of the model, whose primary focus concerns the ability of the individual to care for himself/herself, facilitates its ease of application to the care of the child who has both developmental and health deviation self-care deficits.

The role of the nurse in the care of such children is complex, because there are two foci for that care 'the child' and 'the child's parents/family'. The self-care model provides a very satisfactory framework to explore the nurse's role in detail and also to disentangle the complexities of that role. As discussed above, the role involves both wholly/partially compensatory elements and supportive-educative elements.

The role of the parent is principally that of dependent care agent, but in order for the parent to successfully take on that role, the nurse and other health professionals must both acknowledge and accept the primacy of the parental role and must also take the lead in providing informed support and education to the parents.

The child with asthma has self-care deficits at two levels (developmental and health deviation self care deficits). The self-care model can be usefully employed in identifying the needs of the child arising out of these deficits and also provides a valuable framework for defining the respective roles of parents, nurses and other health professionals as dependent care agents for such a child.

Examples of reading material for children and families

Dyke J (1987). *You Can Do It Desmond Dragon*. Allen and Hanbury's, Greenford, Middlesex.

Hollomby D and Rogan P (1986). *Asthma: The Detective's Story*. Astra Pharmaceuticals, Kings Langley, Hertfordshire.

Wilson R and Pearl K (1983). *Your Child and Asthma*. Astra Pharmaceuticals, Kings Langley, Hertfordshire.

References

Casey A (1988). A partnership with child and family. *Senior Nurse*: **8(4)**: 8–9.

Cleary J, Gray OP, Hall DJ *et al.*(1986). Parental involvement in the lives of children in hospitals. *Archives of Disease in Childhood*; **61**: 779–87.

Henderson V (1964). *Basic Principles of Nursing Care*. International Council of Nurses, Geneva.

Orem DE (1959). *Guides for Developing Curriculum for the Education of Practical Nurses*. U.S. Government Printing Office, Washington D.C.

Orem DE (1971). *Nursing: Concepts of Practice*. McGraw Hill, New York.

Orem DE (1985). *Nursing: Concepts of Practice*. 3rd Edition, McGraw Hill, New York.

Park ES, Golding J, Carswell F *et al.* (1986). Preschool wheezing and prognosis at 10.*Archives of Disease in Childhood*; **61**: 642–6.

Riehl JP and Roy C (1980). *Conceptual Models for Nursing Practice*. Prentice Hall, London.

Roper N, Logan W and Tierney A (1980). *The Elements of Nursing*. Churchill Livingstone, Edinburgh.

Warner JO, Götz M, Landau LI *et al.* (1989). Management of asthma: a consensus statement. *Archives of Disease in Childhood*; **64**: 1065–79.

7

Routine health visiting of a family based upon Becker's health belief model
Yvonne Diment

Introduction

This chapter describes the routine health visiting offered to a family following the birth of their first child, using Becker's health belief model as a framework. The choice of this particular model hinges upon the fact that it attempts to come to terms with the issues of motivation and health behaviour and the weight given to certain influences regarding health decisions.

Description of the model

Hochbaum, Kegeles, Leventhal and Rosenstock (Rosenstock, 1974) originally developed the health belief model based on the social psychological theory of Kurt Lewin (1935). They postulated that the perceived susceptibility of a person to a particular medical condition and the perceived severity of that condition, together with the perceived benefits of action, influenced an individual's state of readiness to engage in a specific health behaviour. The behaviour itself could be triggered by a cue to action which could be either internal or external. Becker *et al.* (1974) introduced the notion of health motivation, that is the degree of interest in and concern about health matters, which in turn was influenced by the perceived susceptibility to an illness, the perceived severity, the benefits or barriers and the cues to action. Modifying factors conditioning perceptions of susceptibility and severity were demographic variables (age, sex etc.)

and sociopsychological variables (reference group pressure, personality, socio-economic status) and cues to action would be interpreted as advice from others (see Figure 7.1).

Research carried out by Kirschst *et al.* (1976) sought to test the model with regard to the advice sought from a local clinic by mothers with a sick child, but they concentrated on behaviour and use of services in the face of illness rather than predicting health-enhancing behaviours incorporated in an everyday lifestyle.

The positive association between perceived severity of a health condition and health behaviour has, however, received increasing support from various research studies. Mikhail (1981) has cited research concerning influenza vaccination, preventive dental visits and use of child health clinics, and Champion (1984) found that the perceived seriousness of the condition of breast cancer was important for regular breast self-examination by women. There is also evidence that 'health consciousness' and concern about health matters is positively correlated with the uptake of prophylactic measures and treatment compliance (Becker *et al.*, 1972; Becker *et al.*, 1977; Becker *et al.*, 1978; Harris and Guten, 1979).

Choice of model

Health visiting is an activity carried out principally with the healthy population as the health visitor's most important function is to promote health and

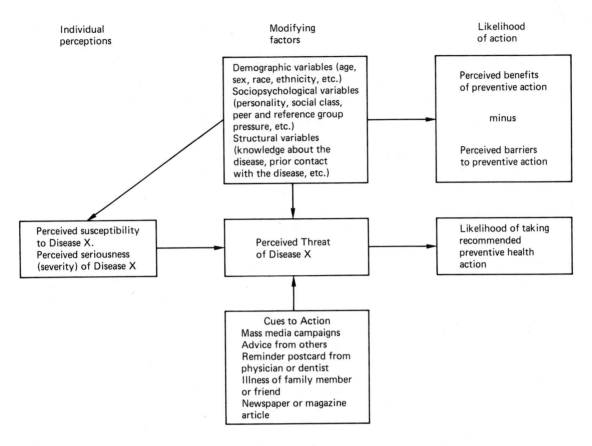

Figure 7.1 The 'health belief model' as a predictor of preventive health behaviour. (Reproduced with permission from Becker *et al.*, 1974, *American Journal of Public Health*; **64(3):** 205–16.)

prevent ill-health (CETHV, 1977). The emphasis is upon working with the client or family and in order to do this effectively it is necessary for communication to be a two-way process. The health belief model allows the health visitor to focus on the client's motivation for acting in a particular way, thus promoting understanding of the client's behaviour. It also emphasizes the process by which health choices are made and the many influences brought to bear in any given situation. The use of a model in this instance was not seen as providing a completely rigid framework, which did not allow for deviation and thus became a strait-jacket, but as a tool to enable certain aspects of the service given to the client to be highlighted. Indeed Coe (1978) has argued that health beliefs are not isolated but intergrated into a complex network of beliefs and values which are part of the culture of any society.

He has thus suggested that any preventive behaviour follows more or less logically from beliefs of the causation of diseases and associated 'appropriate' behaviour. Coe also noted that the health belief model is the only model which incorporates elements of decision-making, together with social and psychological variables. The use of the model is illustrated in the remainder of the chapter by the concentration on three key aspects of health visitor contact with families with young children.

Description of family

This case study describes the health visiting offered to the Lawrence family from the initial visit on the eleventh day following the birth of their first baby,

Individual perceptions	Modifying factors	Likelihood of action
Perceived susceptibility	**Cues for action/barriers**	**Benefits**
Health visitor (DHSS, 1988a)	*Health visitor*	*Health visitor*
Diphtheria – high immunization rate recommended since with minimal naturally occurring infection there is little chance of immunity resulting from sub-clinical infection. Immunization programme must be maintained to combat possible introduction from abroad.	To fulfil function of promoting health and preventing ill-health	Successful completion of immunization programme will prevent or reduce severity of above conditions.
Tetanus – spores found in soil – entry to body via injury or burn.	*Client*	*Client*
Whooping cough – highly infectious. 1975 – safety of vaccine questioned – immunization rate fell from over 80 per cent to approximately 30 per cent – epidemics in 1977/79 and 1981/83.	Sister present at birth visit – her children had both been immunized against diphtheria, tetanus, whooping cough and polio. Client's mother had already advised her to have the injections at the general practitioner's surgery. Louise's father present at fifth visit – had heard that there was concern about one particular injection.	Felt Louise would be 'safer' if she had the immunizations as the conditions must be dangerous, otherwise no injections against them would be offered.
Poliomyelitis – notifications of paralytic poliomyelitis (1976–77) was 25.	*Implementation*	*Costs*
Client	Information concerning immunizations given verbally and in written form at the birth visit. It was noted that Diane wished the injections to be given by the GP. It was assumed by the health visitor that the injection referred to byy Gary was that for whooping cough and the contra-indications were discussed.	Diane is herself anxious about 'needles' and injections and considers them to be painful and is apprehensive about taking Louise for the immunizations as she is unwilling to subject her to pain.
Had not actively considered immunizations. In general discussion it was suggested that 'some people say don't listen to the health visitor.' Reassurance from the client and her sister that they and their mother did not personally subscribe to this. HV reassured client that she was free to accept or reject advice as she deemed appropriate. Louise not felt to be susceptible by client as the criterion used was that nobody in the family had suffered any of the above conditions.	*Evaluation*	
	To monitor the health decisions made by Diane on behalf of Louise.	

Perceived severity

Health visitor (DHSS, 1988a)

Diphtheria – 1979 to 1986 26 cases notified
                                    1 death notified.

Tetanus – 1981 to 1986 – 62 cases notified.

Whooping cough – difficult to estimate number of
                 deaths as the infection is not
                 easily diagnosed.

Side effects – repeated vomiting leading to weight
               loss
             – brain damage.

Poliomyelitis – may result in paralysis.

Client

Uncertain about severity of diphtheria or tetanus
but considered whooping cough to be dangerous
because she had witnessed a case in the son of a
woman for whom she used to babysit and she had
seen at first hand the possible severity of the
condition. Considered polio to be fatal.

Figure 7.2   Infant immunization.

Individual perceptions	Modifying factors	Likelihood of action
Perceived susceptibility	**Cues to action**	**Benefits**
Health visitor	*Health visitor*	*Health visitor*
Louise being bottle-fed. Surveys have found strong links between artificial feeding and early introduction of solids (DHSS, 1988b).	To fulfil function of promoting health and preventing ill-health (CETHV, 1977)	Solids not recommended before three months of age.
Client	*Client*	*Client*
Had not attended antenatal classes but had read books on child care and had first hand knowledge of looking after sister's children.	Baby content. Paternal grandmother had commented that solids could be introduced at two months. Diane said she would have viewed this advice differently if it had come from her own mother but because her boyfriend's mother was older and somewhat old-fashioned, and the manner in which the advice had been offered was interpreted as interfering, then she was not prepared to accept it. Diane concerned that Louise appeared to be constipated at the birth visit – she was adding sugar to the feeds on the advice of her sister and this seemed to be effective.	Louise content on infant formula. Diane felt she could maintain physical contact for longer if she continued with bottle rather than mixed feeding.
Perceived severity	*Implementation*	
Health visitor	Louise weighed weekly and Diane given a record of these weights. Weight gain was within normal limits. Feeding was discussed and Diane supported and reassured concerning Louise's progress. Advice given regarding increasing fluid intake when constipation occurs.	
Case against introduction of solids before 3 months – infant's inability to chew, reluctance to tolerate change of flavour, texture or consistency, vulnerability of gut to infection, predisposition to obesity (DHSS, 1988b).	*Evaluation*	
Client	To monitor when solids introduced.	
Early introduction of solids seen as encouraging Louise to put on weight too rapidly (sister had been advised to wake her child in the night for feeds and was subsequently informed child overweight). Had been told in hospital that introducing solids early could affect the baby's stomach.		

Figure 7.3 Introduction of mixed feeding to infant diet. Overall aim – for Louise to receive a nutritious and appropriate diet.

Individual perceptions	Modifying factors	Likelihood of action
Perceived susceptibility	**Cues to action**	**Benefits**
Health visitor	*Health visitor*	*Health visitor*
Congenital defect-present in a 4–7 per cent of children who come through the perinatal period. Half of these are detected before discharge from hospital (MacFarlane, 1980). Six week check – physical examination including auscultation of heart for early detection of congenital heart disease (Hall, 1989) 6 : 1000 born with congenital heart disease (MacFarlane 1980).	To fulfil function of promoting health and preventing ill-health (CETHV, 1977)	Opportunity for health deficits to be detected and appropriate treatment/support given.
Client	*Client*	*Client*
No specific worries about Louise's health.	Postcard reminder via computerized Child Health System. Verbal reminder from health visitor. Future reference – Diane perceives her sister and her mother as exerting the greatest influence on her with regard to Louise's health. 'Failed' her own hearing test as a child but was subsequently found to have normal hearing. Sister did not take one of her children for routine screening at eight months. This may well have implications as to Diane's decision whether to have Louise's hearing check at eight months. When younger, her sister was prescribed glasses but Diane's father insisted that a second opinion be sought and original diagnosis was subsequently overturned.	Diane attended the local clinic for Louise's six week check with the doctor 'to make sure everything was alright'.
Perceived severity	**Implementation**	
Health visitor	Louise's physical and developmental progress was assessed and a six week check with the clinic doctor offered.	
50 per cent of children and adolescents have 'innocent' heart murmurs (MacFarlane, 1980)	*Evaluation*	
Client	Diane attended the six week check at clinic and a baseline examination was carried out.	
Not considered as Louise appeared healthy.		

Figure 7.4   Routine developmental assessment. Overall aim – to monitor Louise's developmental progress in order that she can realize her full potential.

Louise, to a time when the baby was just over eight weeks old – a total of five visits and four telephone contacts. Diane Lucas, Louise's mother, is unmarried but lives with Louise's father, Gary, and the baby has been given his surname. Diane previously worked as a machinist before she became pregnant and she is also a trained hairdresser. Gary is a plumber and they are currently buying their own home. Diane's mother lives some distance away but her sister and Gary's mother live locally. Louise was born at term plus four days by normal delivery and weighed 3.13 kg.

Immunization was discussed at the initial visit with Diane's sister present and at the fifth visit when Gary and Diane were at home together. As the majority of the visits and contacts involved interaction with Diane as Louise's principal caregiver and the person responsible for her day-to-day care, she is the client referred to in the text (Figure 7.2).

Evaluation of the use of the model

The advantage of using this particular model lies in the fact that it emphasizes the client's perspective of their own or their family's health, and attempts can be made to elicit the reasons for and the influences on an individual's health care decisions. The model thus highlights the fact that the health care professional's contribution is not the only and certainly not the most influential factor in the process of decision-making. In Diane's case she consulted her immediate family for health advice but was also willing to accept that offered by the health visitor. This illustrates the importance of exploring the views already held by the client during the health assessment.

The model can be criticized for focusing too greatly on the individual's responsibility for their own health (the victim-blaming approach) when they may have little or no control over the wider issues which affect their health such as socio-economic status or housing.

However, the model reminds practitioners that they have the potential to facilitate the adoption of preventive health behaviour not only by giving information but also by reducing barriers to the pursuance of such behaviour, for example, by making services 'user-friendly'.

The model, therefore, provides a potential framework towards understanding why some people do or do not pursue preventive health behaviour. However, Rosenstock and Kirscht (1974) acknowledged the model's limitations by stating:

> 'The health belief model is a partially developed theory, many of whose hypotheses have been tested and found useful in explaining behaviour'.
> (p.470)

They did not consider the model complete, but rather as a scientific foundation for the understanding of health behaviour. Indeed, Haefner (1974) referred to the model as an orienting framework to guide both the collection of information and its interpretation, rather than a theory. Interestingly, despite the model's shortcomings, Langlie (1977) has asserted that the health belief model has become the predominant explanation, not only for differences in the use of prophylactic services, but also for differences in preventive health behaviour in general. In the United Kingdom, it is the model most frequently presented to student health visitors and therefore it is regrettable that it has not been subject to extensive testing within the United Kingdom.

References

Becker MH, Drachman RH and Kirscht JP (1972). Predicting mothers' compliance with paediatric medical regimens. *Journal of Pediatrics*; **81**(5): 843–54.

Becker MH, Drachman RH and Kirscht JP (1974). A new approach to explaining sick-role behaviour in low income populations. *American Journal of Public Health*; **64**(3): 205–16.

Becker MH, Nathanson CA, Drachman RH *et al.* (1977). Mother's health beliefs and childrens' clinic visits. *Journal of Community Health*; **3**: 125–35.

Becker MH, Radius SM, Rosenstock IM *et al.* (1978). Compliance with a medical regime for asthma – a test of the Health Belief Model. *Public Health*; **93**: 268–77.

Champion VL (1984). Instrument development for health belief model constructs. *Advances in Nursing Science*; **6**(3): 73–85.

Coe RM (1978). *Sociology of Medicine*. 2nd edition. McGraw-Hill, New York.

Council for the Education and Training of Health Visitors (1977). *An Investigation into the Principles and Practice of Health Visiting*. CETHV London.

Department of Health and Social Security (1988a). *Immunisation against infectious disease*. Joint Committee on Vaccination and Immunisation. London.

DHSS (1988b). *Present Day Practice in Infant Feeding: Third Report*. HMSO, London.

Haefner DP (1974). The health belief model and preventive dental behaviour. *Health Education Monograph*; **2(4)**: 420–32.

Hall DMB (ed) (1989). *Health for all children. Report of the Joint Working Party on Child Health Surveillance*. Oxford University Press, Oxford.

Harris DM and **Guten S** (1979). Health protective behaviour – an exploratory study. *Journal of Health and Social Behaviour*, **20**: 17–29.

Kirschst JP, Becker MH and **Eveland JP** (1976). Psychological and social factors as predictors of medical behaviour. *Medical Care*; **14(5)**: 422–31.

Langlie JK (1977). Social networks, health beliefs and preventive health behaviour. *Journal of Health and Social Behaviour*; **18**: 224–60.

Lewin K (1935). *A Dynamic Theory of Personality*. McGraw-Hill, New York.

MacFarlane JA (1980). *Child Health*. London, Grant McIntyre, Edinburgh.

Mikhail B (1981). The Health Belief Model – a review and critical evaluation of the model, research and practice. *Advances in Nursing Science*; Oct: 65–82.

Rosenstock IM (1974). Historical origins of the Health Belief Model. In Becker MH (ed), *The Health Belief Model and Personal Health Behaviour*. Charles B Slack, New Jersey.

Rosenstock IM and **Kirscht JP** (1974). Practice implications. *Health Education Monograph*; **2(4)**: 470–73.

8

Caring for a child with atopic eczema using Orem's self-care model
Barbara Elliott

Introduction

This chapter describes the use of Orem's self-care model (Orem, 1985) to devise a nursing care plan for Christopher, a three-year-old child admitted to hospital with severe atopic eczema. A brief description of atopic eczema, its incidence, possible causes, associated problems and treatment will be given, followed by a description of the model and reasons for its choice. Orem's model will then be used to make a full assessment of Christopher and his family and plan his care for his stay in hospital. The effectiveness of the nursing care planned and the relevance of Orem's model for paediatric nursing practice will then be evaluated.

Atopic eczema

Atopic eczema is a relatively common skin disease affecting approximately 10 per cent of the British population (Taylor *et al.*, 1984). Prospective studies in England and the United States suggest that the incidence in childhood is five per cent, the majority of children developing the condition in the first year of life (David, 1983).

Atopic eczema is included in the group of atopic diseases which also comprises asthma, allergic rhinitis, allergic conjunctivitis and urticaria. The atopic diseases are frequently familial, however the nature of the genetic predisposition is uncertain. In a study of 75 children with severe atopic eczema, David (1983) found that 90 per cent had a first

degree relative with an atopic disease. As with the other atopic diseases, sufferers of atopic eczema frequently have a raised IgE level, sometimes over 20,000 or 30,000 IU/ml (David, 1983) and these high levels may precede the development of clinical eczema by several months (Hill and Entwisle, 1978). Approximately 60 per cent of children with atopic eczema will go on to develop asthma or allergic rhinitis (David, 1983).

Atopic eczema is characterized by a chronic, pruritic inflammation of the skin, but to refer to it merely as a skin disorder neglects the devastating effect that it can have upon the child and indeed the whole family life. Itching is a major feature of the disease and the need to scratch is overwhelming. Children with severe eczema may lapse into a trance-like state, scratching frantically, apparently oblivious of their surroundings. The damage done to the skin can be considerable and the bleeding and exudation stains clothes and bedding and may cause the materials to stick to the child's skin. The child who is itchy is also usually irritable, and parents and carers are frequently irritated themselves by a child whose behaviour is erratic and uncontrollable and whose constant scratching is deemed to be antisocial and annoying.

Constant itching and discomfort also makes concentration difficult for the child. The child with atopic eczema may have severely restricted resources: walking is difficult with sore, cracked skin around the knees and play is restricted due to sore, cracked hands and poor concentration span, and even eating and laughing prove painful because facial skin is dry and cracks easily. Linked to the itchiness and irritability of children with severe atopic eczema is their inability to sleep. Parents frequently report that their child wakes several times during the night scratching and crying. This not only disrupts the whole family, who may have to develop drastic strategies for coping such as one or both parents sleeping with the child, but then tiredness and exhaustion are added to the problems faced by the child and family the following day.

As with other skin diseases atopic eczema is also disfiguring. The skin is dry and frequently cracked around joints and the lesions are erythematous and lichenified. Such a visible disease, especially on a young child, may cause others to be repulsed and strangers frequently attribute false causes to the condition such as a scald, poor hygiene or infection. This only adds to the child's and parents' feelings of rejection and stress. The social impact of skin diseases is discussed further by Jowett and Ryan (1985).

The cause of atopic eczema is believed to be multifactional. As previously stated, the atopic state is frequently inherited but the actual incidence of the disease is also affected by allergic, dermatological and psychological factors (Faulstich and Williamson, 1985; Ullman *et al.*, 1977; Fergusson *et al.*, 1982). Once the disease is apparent its course and severity is affected by physical factors such as infection (David and Cambridge, 1986); psychological factors (Breton and Latour, 1987); and family environment (Gil *et al.*, 1987). The complex interaction of these factors means that the disease fluctuates dramatically both from child to child and within the same child at different times. The relative importance of each of the factors varies from child to child, so that one child may be mainly affected by allergic factors and another by psychological factors. The suspected pathophysiology of the disease is discussed in depth elsewhere (Sly and Heimlich, 1967).

The complexity of the disease means that no treatment can be approached with any certainty of cure. Indeed, it is recognized that current medical intervention is palliative and only partially effective (Faulstich and Williamson, 1985).

Physical treatments such as topical application of creams and ointments, oral medication and the avoidance of allergens (contact, inhaled, environmental or food) and irritants may be successful, but most sufferers can only hope for some degree of control over their disease rather than cure.

Psychological treatment is not well developed or evaluated, although there have been some encouraging results from the use of hypnotherapy (Glover, 1987) and behaviourally orientated treatment procedures (Cole *et al.*, 1988).

Treatment can prove to be very time-consuming, expensive and sometimes traumatic for the parents of children with atopic eczema. The extra work caused by the disease, such as frequent washing of soiled clothes and bedlinen, is increased by the work generated by treatment. Applying creams and bandages to a screaming, fractious child, constantly providing diversion and play for a child who will scratch if unoccupied or bored, studying food labels for possible allergens, and buying special clothes and bed linen, add to the burden of the disease.

Atopic eczema, therefore, is a very complex disease, which is not merely a skin disorder but which affects almost every aspect of the child's life and consequently the life of the whole family. Furthermore, there is no proven cure for this condition and its severity fluctuates, often for no apparent reason, leaving parents baffled and frustrated. To add to this difficult situation, atopic eczema is frequently misunderstood by outsiders including the medical profession. Atopic eczema is usually non life threatening and undergoes a natural improvement as the child grows older, the majority having outgrown it by the age of twelve. Possibly because of this, eczema is neglected by most of the medical profession and the phrase 'he'll grow out of it', although offered in comfort, frequently causes parents to feel that their child's disease is not being taken seriously (David, 1983).

It is hoped that this brief overview of the disease will give the reader a basic understanding of the condition suffered by Christopher and some of the possible implications for family life.

Selecting a model of nursing

Models have been with us for a very long time. Many nurses view 'nursing models' with at least some degree of fear and trepidation, and yet if they were to think back through their lives they would see that models are as familiar to them as the food that they eat and the clothes they wear. From earliest memory we have played with models – models of cars, trains, babies, houses and used models to make sense of and explain our expanding world. Models represent reality. Some models are very simple representations and some are very complex, aspiring to represent the reality as closely as possible. Models also vary in the degree in which they distort reality, which may be unintentional or on purpose (such as brightly coloured, plastic model ponies with garish pink and green manes).

Nursing models are similarly representations of the reality of nursing practice (MacFarlane, 1986). They identify the components of nursing practice and explain their theoretical basis. They attempt to represent the reality of nursing as closely as possible, but not all models succeed. This may be because the reality as seen by the model's creator does not coincide with that of the person using the model, or occasionally the theoretical basis for the model may be unsound.

Nursing models aim to help those that work with them to understand more fully what they are doing and why they are doing it (Aggleton and Chalmers, 1986). The emphasis is most definitely on help, and nursing models should not make nursing practice more difficult or confusing. Initially, however, using a nursing model may extend our nursing practice, as it may highlight aspects of care which in the past we have tended to ignore. This is particularly relevant as the influence of social and psychological factors upon health and health care are being increasingly recognized. The relationship between such factors should be portrayed by the model of nursing (MacFarlane, 1986) and this is particularly helpful with diseases such as atopic eczema, which are the result of the complex interaction of many such factors.

Given that it is desirable to use a nursing model to guide one's practice, how does one go about selecting an appropriate model? Aggleton and Chalmers (1987) point out that there is a bewildering array of models from which to choose, but caution that choice should be carried out systematically and with care. The nursing model chosen should reflect nurses' and hopefully also patients' views about the nature of people, the nature of nursing, and their concepts of health and the environment.

This is not as simple as it may sound. Nursing education is changing so dramatically at the present time that it is little wonder that the profession contains nurses with widely varying beliefs and values, frequently of a conflicting nature. The theory – practice gap may indeed widen before it is eventually bridged completely. We also live in an increasingly multicultural society, where minority cultures are thankfully being given the respect which they deserve. This however puts nurses in a very difficult position when trying to choose an appropriate model for care. Not only do they have to consider the conflicting beliefs and attitudes of their colleagues about what nursing is or should be about, but they also care for a diverse range of patients both in the type of nursing care that they require and also in *their* beliefs about the sort of nursing they should be given.

We must be wary therefore of imposing models upon nursing staff and patients without some consideration of their individual needs and beliefs. Entire hospitals which use one specific model of nursing should be approached with caution by staff and patients whose value system does not coincide with that of the model. At the very least individual wards should be allowed to choose the model of nursing which reflects the beliefs and values of the majority of staff and the needs of their patients. With increasing use of primary nursing, however, there may be scope for nurses to select the most appropriate model or combination of models for their patients on an individual basis. This would seem a most satisfactory solution.

In selecting a nursing model for the hospital care of a child with atopic eczema a variety of models were considered but after due consideration

Orem's self-care model (Orem, 1985) seemed the most appropriate. Christopher had been cared for successfully by his parents at home despite having a severe, chronic condition. There was no reason to believe that this situation could not be resumed once the exacerbation period of his eczema had passed, and indeed hospital admission was viewed by staff as an opportunity to increase coping and treatment skills for his parents.

There has been a gradual move in recent years to increase the amount of nursing care given to children in hospital by their parents (Webb *et al.*, 1985; Sainsbury *et al.*, 1986). This reflects the changing attitudes of health professionals towards parents and has been seen as desirable by nursing and medical staff as well as parents (Bishop, 1988; Taylor and O'Connor, 1989). Parents are frequently giving technical nursing care such as nasogastric feeds, changing dressings and even giving intravenous drugs (David, 1986). The move towards care-by-parent units, where parents give all the nursing care under the supervision of one nurse, has not been as quickly accepted here as in the States where they originated. One such unit has proved very successful, however, and may be indicative of changes in the future (Cleary *et al.*, 1986).

The trend toward self-care, in terms of patients taking responsibility for their own treatment decisions and moving away from being the passive recipients of medically prescribed therapy, has been evident in diseases such as eczema. Disillusionment with the lack of success of medical treatment and fear of the harmful effects of topical steroids has led many sufferers and parents of sufferers to seek support from self-help organizations such as the National Eczema Society.* Such organizations promote the ideology of self-help whilst offering a balance of mutual support and co-operation.

Orem's self-care model seemed the most suitable choice in light of this situation of increased parental involvement in care, both medically prescribed hospital care and 'alternative' care, and the importance of promoting family independence in

* National Eczema Society, Tavistock House East, Tavistock Square, London WC1H 9SB. Tel: (071) 388 4097.

chronic childhood conditions. Other models such as Roy's stress adaptation model (Roy, 1980) or Roper *et al.* activities of daily living model (1983) would have made a useful contribution to the planning of care, but were not considered to be as consistent with current trends in paediatric nursing.

Orem's self-care model

Nursing models are classified according to their primary focus or theory. The three main categories of models are interactionist models, systems models and developmental models.

There is some debate in the literature about the category into which Orem's self-care model fits. Riehl and Roy (1980) refer to Orem's model as a systems model and indeed Orem (1985) does refer to nursing systems. As Webb (1986) points out, however, the term is not developed in line with general systems theory in terms of input, output and feedback. Fawcett (1984) classifies the self-care model as being a developmental model and indeed developmental theory has a strong influence in that Orem (1985) recognizes that there are developmental self-care requisites and that a person's position on the developmental continuum will determine his ability for self-care. Probably the most satisfactory classification is that by Thibodeau (1983) who refers to Orem's model as an eclectic model, i.e. one that uses two or more types of theory as its theoretical base. Thibodeau (1983) recognizes that there is equal emphasis upon concepts from developmental, interactionist and systems theories in Orem's model.

Orem (1985) defines self care as:

'The production of actions directed to self or to the environment in order to regulate one's functioning in the interest of one's life, integrated functioning and well-being.'

(p.31)

Orem (1985) recognizes that not all persons are able to give their own self-care, notably children, and that they depend on others, usually their parents, to give the required care which Orem calls dependent care.

The need for nursing care arises when a person's ability for self-care or care of dependents is limited by the health situations of the recipients of care (Orem, 1985). The focus of nursing is on the individual and their unique needs. In the case of nursing children, the self-care model recognizes that the dependent care agent (usually the parents) are the most suitable people to give care to the child and that nursing should aim towards that end.

Orem (1985) does, however, recognize that self-care and care of dependents may be well intentioned, but not always therapeutic. The nurse must determine the therapeutic value of practices prescribed by a patient's general culture or by other health professionals. This is particularly important in atopic eczema where, in desperation for help, parents may seek advice from lay people (grandparents, friends and even people on the street often have an opinion to offer on how to treat a rash). Alternative therapies such as homeopathic medicine are also used. Such advice may or may not be helpful and the nurse must enable the parents to assess its therapeutic value. At the same time the nurse must be wary of imposing her own beliefs on patients if they are in conflict with the values and beliefs of the patient's culture. Emphasis must be on assessing the therapeutic value of care as perceived by the patient.

Assessment

Orem does not actually refer to the assessment phase of the nursing process as such, but rather the elements of diagnosis. This involves calculation of the therapeutic self- or dependent-care demand and assessment of the self- or dependent-care agency including potential for self- or dependent-care agency in the future. In health there should be an equal balance between these two.

Orem (1985) defines the therapeutic self-care demand as:

'the measures of care required at moments in time in order to meet existent requisites for regulatory action to maintain life and to maintain or promote health and development and general well being'.

(p.31)

Self- or dependent-care agency is the ability to perform self- or dependent-care. The dependent-care agent is the provider of care for infants, children or dependent adults. In this society it is usually the mother of the family.

If the therapeutic dependent care demands exceed the dependent-care abilities there exists a dependent-care deficit. The nurse must then determine the qualitative or quantitative inadequacy of the dependent-care agency and determine the nature and reasons for the dependent-care deficit. This will enable the nurse to decide on the appropriate nursing systems to enable the family to return to a state of dependent care.

It should be noted that the dependent-care deficit may be due to an increase in dependent-care demands or a decrease in dependent-care abilities, or both. The complex skills required to balance the needs of a family with the resources available to her will be familiar to most mothers. Even a slight increase in demand on her overstretched resources may result in an inability to cope at all.

Orem (1985) acknowledges that deficits in self-care or dependent-care may arise from the composition and complexity of the therapeutic self- or dependent-care demands as well as from the health of developmental states of the recipients of care. Calculation of the therapeutic self-care or dependent-care demand involves assessment of three categories of self-care requisites, specified by Orem (1985). These are universal self-care requisites which are common to all human beings and are associated with life processes; self-care requisites which are related to the developmental stage of the individual and the effects on that development of environmental factors; and health deviation self-care requisites, which arise out of ill health. There then follows identification of factors which will affect the way in which each self-care requisite can be met and identification of the interrelationship between the different categories of self care requisites. Courses of action to meet the various self- or dependent- care requisites must then be designed.

Having calculated the patient's therapeutic self-care demand, the nurse must then make an assessment of the self-care or dependent-care agency, that is the ability of the patient or his carer to meet these demands. Orem (1985) warns that this determination of the abilities of an individual to engage in self- or dependent-care must be accurately carried out otherwise:

'nurses have no rational basis for:
1. making judgments about existing or projected self-care deficits and the reasons for their existence;
2. selecting valid and reliable methods of helping or
3. prescribing and designing nursing systems'.
(p.107)

This indeed is the next step in the process – deciding where a dependent- or self-care deficit exists and planning with the patient and family how to remove this deficit. This may be achieved by decreasing the dependent- or self-care demands, increasing the dependent- or self-care abilities or the nurse meeting the demands directly herself.

Planning care

The self-care deficits form the problem statements for the care plan and the overall goal of nursing care must be the elimination of the self-care deficits (Pearson and Vaughan, 1985). Orem (1985) recognizes that the nurse has three basic variations in nursing systems to allow her to achieve this goal.

- Wholly compensatory nursing systems.
- Partly compensatory nursing systems.
- Supportive – educative (developmental) nursing systems.

In the case of a child, the nurse must ask herself who should be meeting the therapeutic self-care demands; the child himself, the mother or other relative as dependent-care agent, or the nurse. Orem (1985) also describes five methods of helping from which the nurse can choose when planning her patients care.

- Doing for or acting for another.
- Guiding and directing another.
- Providing physical or psychological support.
- Providing an environment that supports development.
- Teaching.

Christopher Brown's admission to hospital

Christopher is a three-year-old boy who was diagnosed as suffering from atopic eczema when he was six months old. He has been treated for this condition by the family general practitioner and by a local dermatologist as an outpatient.

Christopher's parents coped with his prescribed treatment at home until May 1989 when his skin deteriorated markedly over the Bank Holiday weekend. They were not satisfied with the attitude of or treatment prescribed by the on-call family doctor and so took Christopher to the accident and emergency department of the local children's hospital. Here he was seen by the medical registrar who admitted him to one of the medical wards.

On arrival on the ward, information was collected in order to determine Christopher's need for nursing care. This was obtained from his parents, who accompanied him to the ward, Christopher himself, his medical notes and other members of the health care team.

Christopher's mother expressed a desire to be resident on the ward because 'he can be very fretful and he needs so much special care'.

His five year old brother, John, and eight year old sister, Elizabeth, would be cared for by maternal grandparents who were already staying wih the family for the holiday break. Christopher's father would visit each evening after work.

The following assessment of Christopher and his family was made during the first few days of his admission to hospital (Figure 8.1). Orem (1985) sees assessment as a continuous process and indeed the depth of information required by the model could not be obtained in a one-off admission interview. Rather Christopher's primary nurse gathered the information over several days as her

Therapeutic self- or dependent-care demand	Current self- or dependent-care agency	Self- or dependent-care deficit	Future potential for self- or dependent-care
A: *Universal self-care requisites* 1. Maintenance of sufficient intake of air.			
C – breathe normally unassisted	C – colour good, respiratory rate 27 per min.	C – None	
P – recognize realistic risk of developing asthma and recognize signs and symptoms of onset.	P – very anxious that C will develop asthma as father suffered severely as a child.	P – knowledge deficit regarding inheritance of atopic diseases and signs and symptoms of asthma.	P – with adequate information anxiety should be more realistic.
2. Maintenance of sufficient intake of water.			
C – drink a variety of fluids as desired	C – can indicate his desire for drink verbally but cannot pour one himself. Cannot discriminate between permitted and non-permitted drinks.	C – skills deficit. Requires drinks provided by persons aware of restrictions.	C – cannot be self caring due to stage development.
P – ensure that C drinks approximately 1.5 litres fluid/day. Avoiding cow's milk and any drinks containing artificial colours or preservatives as these are known to exacerbate his eczema.	P – fully aware of restrictions but unsure of available drinks in hospital.	P – knowledge deficit of available drinks on ward.	P – with appropriate information will be able to provide dependent care.
3. Maintenance of sufficient intake of food.			
C – eat well balanced diet within restrictions.	C – appetite good wt = 35 lbs. Tends to cheat on diet and wants to eat same food as siblings.	C – knowledge and motivation deficit.	C – cannot be self-caring due to stage of development, but may respond to explanation and reward for good behaviour.
P – ensure C eats a nutritious diet avoiding eggs, dairy produce, fish, artificial colours and preservatives.	P – able to purchase and prepare suitable food. Avoid all convenience foods. Considering putting whole family on restricted diet to avoid conflict.	P – some knowledge deficit regarding variety of suitable foods.	P – with increased knowledge and coping skills will be able to give dependent care.

4. Provision of care associated with elimination. C – alert carers of need to eliminate in sufficient time. P – supervise C to prevent skin damage and monitor care of clothes and environment.	C – asks for 'wee' or 'potty'. Able to use adult toilet with assistance. Excoriated skin causes pain on micturition so tries to avoid until last minute, scratches exposed skin when using toilet. Bowels open once/day. Soft stool. P – aware of signs that C may need to urinate and of need to supervise to prevent excessive scratching.	C – reluctant to pass urine because of pain. Unable to control urge to scratch when skin exposed. P – None	C – if pain reduced should be more willing to pass urine. Unlikely to be able to control urge to scratch whilst eczema present.
5. Maintenance of balance between activity and rest. C – play appropriately for age and stage of development. Rest and sleep sufficiently for recuperation. P – provide stimulating activities to prevent boredom avoiding substances which may exacerbate eczema. Provide suitable environment for sleep and rest.	C – enjoys Lego, drawing and energetic games. Concentration span limited and easily frustrated. Eczema on hands and legs limits dexterity and ability through pain. Bedtime 8pm. Wakes 3–4 times each night scratching. P – exhausted by constant need to occupy C and lack of sleep.	C – skills deficit due to pain and poor concentration. Unable to sleep through night. P – knowledge deficit regarding suitable toys and games. Support deficit.	C – skills should improve with improvement in skin condition. May develop better sleeping pattern. P – Need to be relieved of some dependent care to improve coping ability.
6. Maintenance of balance between solitude and social interaction. C – develop social skills appropriate for age. P – enable C to develop social contacts with peers and gain independence.	C – enjoys playing with siblings, but has few friends. P – take C to nursery two mornings/week. Eczema always worse on return so considering stopping. Do not allow C to play at other children's houses for fear of effect of pets or dust on skin.	C – social development limited by lack of interaction with peers. P – knowledge deficit regarding importance of social development and minimising isolation.	C – potential for normal social development with increased interactions with peers. P – may achieve more appropriate balance with increased knowledge.

Figure 8.1 Assessment of Christopher and his family. (C = Christopher, P = parents).

Therapeutic self- or dependent-care demand	Current self- or dependent-care agency	Self- or dependent-care deficit	Future potential for self- or dependent-care
7. Prevention of hazards to human life, functioning and well being. C – gain knowledge of potential hazards appropriate to age. P – be aware of usual hazards for 3 year old children and factors particularly hazardous to C's eczema. Avoid or control such hazards and minimise harmful effects.	C – unaware of potential hazards, lacks sense of danger and is inquisitive and adventurous. P – aware of potential hazards and particular risk to C from certain foods, house dust mites, animal fur and dander. Refused immunizations because of eczema. Had experience of severe allergic reaction and aware of signs and symptoms and appropriate action.	C – knowledge and motivation deficit appropriate for age. P – knowledge deficit regarding immunizations.	C – should learn hazards to be avoided with increasing age and cognitive ability. P – well motivated to learn if accurate information provided.
8. Being normal. C – realistic self-image and identification with peers. P – as far as possible minimize C's feelings of being different and promote a positive self-image.	C – refused to wear shorts this summer as feels his legs look 'horrid'. Dad heard some children calling C 'Scabby'. P – believe that C's eczema must take priority and C must be protected from harmful factors. Mum believes people think she does not care for C properly as he looks dirty.	C – becoming aware that he does not look 'normal' but lacks understanding of why. P – unable to promote positive self image when acutely aware of own negative image as parents.	C – feelings of abnormality should be minimized by stressing positive aspects of image. P – with increased support and understanding may be able to offer dependent-care.

B. Developmental self-care requisites			
B. Developmental self-care requisites Bring about and maintain living conditions that support life and promote development. Prevent or overcome the harmful effects of conditions that can effect development.	C – Gross motor skills, can run, climb, ride tricycle but abilities limited by pain when eczema severe. Fine motor skills limited by pain due to swollen, inflamed and broken skin on hands. Development delayed due to periods of having hands bandaged. Social development and play – friendly boy, used to adult company and having his own way. Hearing and speech – vocabulary good. Using short sentences. Hearing tests passed.	C – motor skills deficit. Limited social skills. Unwilling to share or take turns as used to being given in to. Cries and scratches when frustrated.	C – motor skills should improve with improved skin condition. Social skills may improve with increased contact with peers.
C – achieve appropriate development milestones and develop identity as son, brother, and friend. Accept some lasting dependence on carers due to eczema.			
P – provide stimulating and safe environment to allow C to develop fully within limitations of disease.	P – aware that some aspects of development delayed due to restrictions of eczema. Believe C will catch up once cured.	P – motivation deficit to promote development as fear deterioration of skin. Knowledge deficit regarding long term nature of eczema.	P – with more information may be able to achieve better balance between developmental needs and care of eczema.

Figure 8.1 Continued. (C = Christopher, P = parents).

Therapeutic self- or dependent-care demand	Current self- or dependent-care agency	Self- or dependent-care deficit	Future potential for self- or dependent-care
C. *Health deviation self-care requisites* 1. Seek and secure appropriate medical assistance. P – request help from medical and nursing staff as needed.	P – disillusioned with medical care after 2½ years of unsuccessful treatment. Relieved that C admitted to hospital and disease taken seriously.	P – lack of confidence in medically prescribed treatment. Potential for non-compliance.	P – confidence may be restored with understanding and reassurance.
2. Be aware of and attend to the effects of pathological states. C – inform carers if skin feels dry, hot, painful or itchy and co-operate with treatment. P – be alert to signs of deterioration in C's skin or behaviour and treat appropriately. Be aware of and deal with effects of eczema on other family members.	C – behaviour indicates deterioration in skin – scratching, irritability. P – aware of signs of deterioration. Limited ability to treat. Aware that other children do not get as much attention as C and parents are irritable with each other.	C – cannot verbalize feelings yet. Refuses to cooperate with treatment due to fear and stage of development. P – skills deficit in treating eczema effectively through fear of distressing C further. Support deficit.	C – fear will be reduced if learns that treatment can be soothing. P – need relief from care until C more cooperative. Support may provide more energy for other family members.
3. Effectively carry out medically prescribed measures. C – co-operate with treatment. P – consistently carry out treatment for prescribed period.	C – screams when any creams applied, refuses to take medication. P – upset by C's behaviour and fear hurting him so often omit treatment. Doubt effectiveness of treatment.	C – as above. P – skills deficit as above. Motivation deficit.	C – as above. P – need relief from care as above. Evidence of therapeutic value should increase motivation to persist with treatment.
4. Be aware of attend to side-effects of medical care. C – inform carers if feels unwell. P – be alert to possible side-effects of restricted diets, topical steroids, sedatives or other prescribed treatment.	C – limited ability to verbalize feelings, but behaviour will indicate health state. P – little knowledge of side-effects except those of steroids.	C – none P – knowledge deficit.	P – if information provided, well motivated to observe and report side effects.

5. Modify self-concept to accept oneself as being in a particular state of health and in need of specific health care.	C – becoming aware that he has eczema, but unable to associate skin state with treatment.	C – unable to understand disease therefore acceptance limited.	C – as cognitive ability develops will learn cause and effect nature of disease.
C – accept and cooperate with treatment and restrictions.			
P – accept chronic nature of eczema, but modify concept of C as being very sick.	P – believe that C can be cured.	P – knowledge deficit regarding chronic nature of eczema. Motivation deficit.	P – may be unable to accept possibility of no cure.
6. Learn to live with effects of pathological conditions and medical treatment measures in a lifestyle which promotes continued personal development.	C – some acceptance of eczema, but not of treatment.	C – will not tolerate treatment.	C – may accept treatment if he can associate with feeling better.
C – accept eczema and treatment.			
P – incorporate care of C into a normal and satisfying lifestyle.	P – family life dominated by care of C's eczema. Parents tired and irritable. Other children 'play up' when feel neglected.	P – knowledge deficit. Skills deficit and support deficit.	P – will need much support and more co-operation from C to improve quality of life.

Figure 8.1 Continued. (C = Christopher, P = parents).

Self, or dependent care deficit	Self or dependent care goal	Nursing intervention
1. Parents lack knowledge regarding the risk of C developing asthma.	Parents will have accurate information regarding asthma.	i) Provide accurate up to date information (verbal and written) about incidence of asthma in children with eczema = T ii) Encourage parents to discuss anxieties with medical staff and ask questions = G iii) Provide verbal and written information regarding signs and symptoms of onset of asthma = T iv) Encourage parents to contact GP or hospital if concerned about C's breathing = G
2. C is unable to provide himself with drinks when thirsty. Parents unaware of suitable drinks available for C.	C will have drinks as desired which comply with dietary restrictions.	i) Ensure all nursing, play and medical staff are aware of restricted diet and fluids = E ii) Offer C suitable drinks with other children and encourage him to ask for drinks as desired = D iii) Show parents where they can prepare and store C's drinks = T
3. C is reluctant to adhere to restricted diet. Parents lack knowledge and skills to enforce restricted diet.	C will only eat permitted foods. Parents will be more confident in enforcing diet.	i) As in 2(i) ii) Refer parents to dietician = E and T iii) Encourage C to share mealtimes with other children, explaining why his meals are special = S and E iv) Reserve one or two favourite foods as treats to reward good behaviour = S v) Encourage parents to praise good behaviour at meal times = G
4. C is reluctant to pass urine due to pain which leads to 'accidents'. Scratches exposed skin when using the toilet.	Reduced/eliminated pain. Minimal skin damage.	i) Apply treatment as prescribed = D ii) Obtain urine specimen for laboratory analysis to detect possible infection = D iii) Ask C if he needs to 'wee' hourly, encourage parents to do the same = D and G iv) Supervise C using toilet if parents unavailable. Distract to discourage scratching = S v) Observe for signs of increased or decreased pain. Ask parents to report same = D and G
5. C is unable to play unsupervised. Tired due to night-time waking. Parents lack knowledge regarding suitable games and activities. Tired due to lack of sleep and support.	C will have suitable play activities to promote development and to prevent boredom. P will have adequate knowledge and support to provide above. Family will have improved sleeping pattern.	i) Involve play therapist and parents in preparing an activity programme for C balancing energetic and quiet play and promoting development of motor and social skills = T and E ii) Involve medical staff and parents in compiling a list of toys and activities to be avoided due to detrimental effect on eczema eg. sand play, water play and furry toys = T and E iii) Encourage parents to take breaks whilst C is playing with play therapist and other children to increase his independence and their rest = S and E. iv) Encourage other family members (siblings, grandparents) to be involved in play programme so that they can support parents after discharge = G and E v) Promote improved sleep pattern through treatment

Problem	Goal	Nursing action
6. C has limited social interaction with peers, because of parental fear of deterioration of eczema and lack of knowledge.	C will develop social skills through increased contact with peers. Parents fear will be reduced to manageable level.	i) Encourage parents to voice fears and discuss ways of minimising risks outside the home – eg. contact play group to discuss C's social needs, provide play group leader with copies of play programme and diet sheet = S and G ii) Provide parents with information regarding the importance of social development = T iii) Contact local branch of National Eczema Society who may provide parents with names of local families to offer support = E
7. C is unaware of hazards in environment both general and specific to his eczema. P lack current information regarding immunisations.	C will avoid hazards. Parents will gain knowledge and make informed decision regarding immunizations.	i) Ensure C is supervised when parents not present on ward = D ii) Ensure all staff aware of hazards to C's eczema and signs and symptoms of adverse reaction = E iii) Ask consultant to discuss immunizations with parents = G
8. C unable to understand why skin appears different to other children. Parents unable to promote a normal self-image.	C will accept his eczema and develop a positive self image.	i) Encourage parents to discuss their feelings about C's appearance and the reaction of others to it = S ii) Discuss methods of promoting a positive self image through clothes and praise = G and T iii) Encourage contact with other affected families to share ideas and offer support = E iv) Explain to C that he has eczema and that is not his fault. Stress his positive features and encourage parents to do the same = S and T
9. C has limited motor skills due to pain from eczema and treatment of eczema and undeveloped social skills. Parents lack knowledge regarding long term nature of eczema and importance of promoting normal development.	C will reach expected developmental milestones within two months (review in one month).	i) Develop play programmes as in 5 to promote development of deficient skills. Promote social contact as in 6 ii) Treat eczema as prescribed to reduce pain and increase movement. (If bandages prescribed, only apply at night time) = D iii) Medical staff to discuss with parents realistic expectations of control of eczema rather than complete cure. Encourage parents to ask questions and discuss their anxieties and expectations = T and G iv) Provide information regarding normal child development and how this may be effected by eczema and methods of minimising effects = T
10. Parents lack confidence in medically prescribed treatment of eczema.	Parents will regain confidence whilst recognizing 'trial and error' nature of many treatments.	i) Encourage parents to discuss treatment with consultant and agree mutually acceptable trial periods = G ii) Treatment only to be given by primary nurse parents and associate nurse to enable C to develop trust in nurses and aid assessment of improvement or deterioration of eczema = D and S

Figure 8.2 Christopher's care plan. (D = doing for another, S = providing support, E = providing supportive environment, G = guiding another, T = teaching).

Self, or dependent care deficit	Self or dependent care goal	Nursing intervention
11. C is reluctant to co-operate with treatment due to fear. Parents lack skills in dealing with behaviour and therefore motivation to continue with treatment.	C will co-operate with treatment. Parents will be able to give effective treatment within 4 days.	i) Primary (or associate) nurse to apply creams, file nails and give oral medication as prescribed for first two days, to relieve parents of stress of treatment and to act as a role model = D ii) Parents to resume treatment with assistance and support from primary nurse as they feel confident = S iii) Incorporate play and involve C in applying creams = S iv) Avoid if possible, creams that genuinely sting and through gentle but firm insistence show C that he need not fear pain = S and T v) Explain all treatment to C before commencing and where possible show him what to expect = T vi) Reward C after treatment and praise good, co-operative behaviour = S
12. Parents lack knowledge regarding possible side effects of treatment.	Parents will demonstrate verbally adequate knowledge before discharge.	i) Parent to discuss current knowledge with Primary nurse to identify deficiencies = G ii) Involve medical staff and dietician in providing accurate information regarding possible side effects = T iii) Ensure parents have out patient appointment and contact number on discharge and encourage contact if concerned about any aspect of treatment = S
13. C has limited understanding of eczema and thus limited acceptance.	As C's cognitive ability increases he will show increasing understanding and acceptance of disease and treatment.	i) Encourage parents to explain eczema and treatment (including dietary restrictions) to C. Use books and pictures to help explanations = G and T ii) Praise C when his skin is improving and encourage him to link improvement with his actions = T and S iii) Introduce C to other children with eczema = E
14. Family life dominated by C's eczema and treatment.	Family will develop a more satisfying lifestyle incorporating C's care.	i) Encourage parents to develop more realistic expectations as in 9. ii) Encourage positive image of C as in 8. iii) Assess need for formal counselling and refer as necessary (review in 1 month at out patient appointment) = E iv) Involve other family members in care during admission (grandparents and siblings) and encourage parents to continue after discharge = E v) Encourage contact with other families with eczema = E

Figure 8.2 Continued. (D = doing for another, G = guiding another, S = providing support, E = providing supportive environment. T = teaching).

relationship with Christopher and his family developed. A system of primary nursing is used on the ward to which Christopher was admitted. The scope of this chapter does not allow for a discussion of primary nursing, but the reader is referred to sources such as Manthey (1980) and Giovannetti (1986).

Evaluation

Nurses writing about models have repeatedly challenged practising nurses to evaluate the pertinence of various models to their work situation and critically analyse their effectiveness (MacFarlane, 1986; Aggleton and Chalmers, 1986). Nursing models may have been created in ivory towers, but their usefulness and credibility stands or falls with the practising nurse involved in the direct delivery of nursing care. If a model cannot be used or adapted to the particular needs of the clinical situation then it will sit upon the book shelves forever.

Orem's self-care model proved useful in assessing Christopher and his family and their abilities for self- and dependent-care. Possibly due to the complex nature of a disease such as eczema and its impact upon so many aspects of a sufferer's life, the assessment proved rather lengthy. It was important that the assessment process continued over the whole of Christopher's admission to hospital, as information regarding some aspects of parental knowledge was only discovered towards the end of his hospital stay. In light of this it is important that the same nurse assesses, plans and delivers care for several days, preferably during the whole admission, so that she has an opportunity to build up her knowledge of the family and develop a therapeutic relationship with them.

The special consideration of developmental self-care requisites proved beneficial in caring for a child whose developmental stage may be affected by his disease, admission to hospital or both. The detailed assessment of health deviation self-care requisites proved to be most enlightening. Attitudes towards health care and abilities to carry out prescribed treatment are often not fully assessed. It is frequently assumed that patients or their families will actively seek medical help as needed and co-operate unquestioningly with prescribed treatment. In a disease such as eczema, where treatment is not always successful, it is important that the nurse recognizes that there may be barriers to compliance and the cost of treatment in terms of emotional strain and family conflict may outweigh the often doubtful benefits.

The assessment also highlighted the connections between problems or care-deficits. For example, the self- and dependent-care deficits relating to 'being normal' and developmental requisites were closely related to the family's ability to live with the effects of eczema and its treatment in a lifestyle which promoted continued personal development.

Devising the plan of care for Christopher and his parents proved interesting as the respective roles of the nurses and Christopher's parents had to be negotiated for each problem. After two and a half years of delivering dependent-care with very little support it was important that the nurse did not completely take over Christopher's care. Rather she had to discuss with his parents those aspects of care with which they wished to have help and tactfully suggest those aspects with which the medical and nursing staff considered that they required aid. For some problems, such as applying creams and administering oral medications, the parents were relieved to temporarily relinquish care to a nurse, but with other problems such as those associated with play and development, it was more difficult for Christopher's parents to accept their limitations and need for professional guidance. The negotiation of roles in caring for sick children in hospital is being given increasing consideration, with nurses realizing that parents have important skills to offer. Thus Orem's model is useful in illustrating the negotiation process and encouraging the involvement of family in care.

The inter-relationship between problems led to some repetition in the care plan and it was necessary to cross-reference prescribed care. In practice this could be reduced by condensing the care plan. The potential for conflict between self-care goals for Christopher and dependent-care goals for his parents was recognized, but did not in fact arise. Chronically ill children aspiring towards independence are frequently in conflict with parents, who tend to be over-protective. It is important therefore that the model of choice acknowledges the different priorities of the patient, family carers and nurses, so as to address this potential conflict directly.

The nature of chronic diseases such as eczema inevitably means that evaluation of planned care is an ongoing process. The goals for some of the problems were necessarily long-term and could not be fully evaluated by the time Christopher was discharged. Ideally follow-up at out-patient clinic would involve the primary nurse so that evaluation could be continued and goals modified according to progress.

Conclusion

Orem's model has been used extensively in the United States with some considerable success (Fawcett, 1984). It has also been demonstrated that nurses taught with a curriculum based upon Orem's self-care deficit theory are likely to continue to use this theory and adapt it to their practice after graduation (Wagnild et al., 1987). There are, however, some problems with the concept of self-care and the application of Orem's model in all situations. The multi-cultural society existing in Britain today has already been mentioned as a factor to be considered when choosing a model of nursing. Self-care may not be a valid concept in all cultures and indeed the traditional view of health care in the UK is that patients are admitted to hospital to be cared for.

Having contributed towards the National Health Service patients see it as their right to be given skilful, sympathetic care by nurses who are not going to suggest that they 'do it themselves' at the earliest opportunity. Even though it has been suggested that increased participation of parents in the care of their sick child in hospital is desirable, this may not always be so. Parents giving continuous dependent care to a chronically ill child may value his admission to hospital as a respite from the work of caring and be only too glad to relinquish dependent-care to others. Nurses adopting a self-care model must be wary of implying that good parents want to care for their sick children and those who do not are negligent. Fear of being

labelled as negligent may prevent parents from admitting that they need a break and nurses should be prepared to care in a wholly compensatory manner for as long as necessary.

The other major reservation about Orem's self-care model is the definition of persons with a legitimate need for nursing. Such persons are characterized:

'a) by a demand for discernible kinds and amounts of self-care or dependent-care and b) by health-derived or health-related limitations for the continuing production of the amount and kind of care required. In dependent-care situations the limitations of dependent care givers are associated with the health state and the care requirements of the dependent person'.
(Orem, 1985, p.30)

This description of dependent-care limited by the health state and care requirements of the dependent person seems to be over-simplified and not necessarily descriptive of the situation with chronically ill children. Parents, and particularly mothers, often have several persons requiring dependent-care from them, not only their children but elderly relatives, neighbours and spouses. Their resources and dependent-care abilities have to be shared and balanced between the demands from these different sources. A deficit between the dependent-care demanded by a chronically sick child and the dependent-care ability of the mother may well be due to a deterioration in the child's health, but could equally be caused by illness in another dependent or loss of her partners support through separation or divorce. It is true that these latter situations would not justify nursing care in the strictest sense; however, it is a reality that children are admitted to hospital for 'social reasons and not just health-related problems. This may be viewed as a form of prevention, certainly in diseases such as eczema where family stresses may soon lead to a deterioration of the disease, and early intervention in terms of support or respite care may well prevent the child needing far more extensive treatment and care in the future.

Despite these criticisms the self-care model developed by Orem would appear to have much to offer paediatric nursing and care of the chronically ill. It may have been somewhat ahead of its time, but the philosophy of individuals being responsible for their own health and that of dependents has become more acceptable in recent years and is in keeping with the political persuasion of the 1990s. Like all nursing models it is only a partial representation of reality, and it should be used only with careful thought.

References

Aggleton P and **Chalmers H** (1986). *Nursing Models and the Nursing Process.* Macmillan Education Ltd., Basingstoke.

Aggleton P and **Chalmers H** (1987). Models of nursing practice and nurse education. *Journal of Advanced Nursing*; **12**: 573–81.

Bishop J (1988). Sharing the caring. *Nursing Times*; **84**(33): 60–1.

Breton JJ and **Latour R** (1987). Pediatric psychiatry and dermatology: presentation of a case of atopic dermatitis. *Canadian Journal of Psychiatry*, **32**(5): 395–8.

Cole WC, Roth HL and **Sachs LB** (1988). Group psychotherapy as an aid in the medical treatment of eczema. *Journal of American Academy of Dermatology*; **18**: 286–91.

Cleary J, Grey OP, Hall DJ et al., (1986). Parent involvement in the lives of children in hospitals. *Archives of Disease in Childhood*; **61**: 770–87.

David TJ (1983). The investigation and treatment of severe eczema in childhood. *International Medicine Supplement*; **6**: 17–25.

David TJ (1986). *Cystic Fibrosis in Children. Practical and Legal Aspects of Intravenous Antibiotic Administration in the home.* Excerpta Medica, Amsterdam.

David TJ and **Cambridge GC** (1986). Bacterial infection and atopic eczema. *Archives of Disease in Childhood*; **61**: 20–3.

Faulstich ME and **Williamson DA** (1985). An overview of atopic dermatitis: toward a bio-behavioural integration. *Journal of Psychosomatic Research*; **29**(6): 647–54.

Fawcett J (1984). *Analysis and Evaluation of Conceptual Models of Nursing*, F.A. Davis Company, Philadelphia.

Fergusson DM, Horwood LJ, Shannon FT (1982). Risk factors in childhood eczema. *Journal of Epidemiology and Community Health*; **36**(2): 118–22.

Gil KM, Keefe FJ, Sampson HA et al. (1987). The relation of stress and family environment to atopic dermatitis symptoms in children. *Journal of Psychosomatic Research*; **31**(6): 673–84.

Giovannetti P (1986). Evaluation of primary nursing, in Weilty HH, Fitpatrick JJ, Taunton RL (eds) *Annual Review of Nursing Research.* Springer Publishing Co., New York.

Glover M (1987). Hypnosis – a useful treatment for eczema. *Exchange*; **47**: 4–5.

Hill D and **Entwisle B** (1978). Atopic eczema and allergy in early childhood. *Medical Journal of Australia*, Special Supplement; **Dec**: 7–8.

Jowett S and **Ryan T** (1985). Skin disease and handicap: an analysis of the impact of skin conditions. *Social Science and Medicine*; **20 4**: 425–9.

MacFarlane J (1986). The value of models for care, in Kershaw B and Salvage J (eds), *Models for Nursing.* John Wiley, Chichester.

Manthey M (1980). *The Practice of Primary Nursing.* Blackwell, Oxford.

Orem DE (1985). *Nursing: Concepts of Practice* 3rd Ed. McGraw-Hill Book Company, New York.

Pearson A and **Vaughan B (1986)**. *Nursing Models for Practice.* Heinemann Nursing, London.

Riehl J and **Roy C** (eds) (1980). *Conceptual Models for Nursing Practice.* Appleton-Century-Crofts, New York.

Roper L, Logan WW and **Tierney AJ** (1983). *Using a Model of Nursing.* Churchill Livingstone, Edinburgh.

Roy C (1980). The Roy Adaptation Model, in Riehl J and Roy C (Eds), *Conceptual Models for Nursing Practice.* Appleton-Century-Crofts, New York.

Sainsbury CPQ, Gray OP, Cleary J et al. (1986). Care by parents of their children in hospital. *Archives of Disease in Childhood*; **61**: 612–15.

Sly RM and **Heimlich EM** (1967). Physiologic abnormalities in the atopic state: a review. *Annals of Allergy*; **25**: 192–210.

Taylor B, Wadsworth M, Wadsworth J et al. (1984). Changes in the reported prevalence of childhood eczema since 1939–45 war. *Lancet*; **1st Dec**: 1255–7.

Taylor MRH and **O'Connor P** (1989). Resident parents and shorter hospital stay. *Archives of Diseases in Childhood*; **64**(2): 274–6.

Thibodeau JA (1983). *Nursing Models; Analysis and Evaluation.* Wadsworth Health Sciences Division, California.

Ullman KC, Moore RW and **Reidy M** (1977). Atopic eczema, A clinical psychiatric study. *Journal of Asthma Research*; **14**(2): 91–9.

Wagnild G, Rodriguez W and **Pritchett G** (1987). Orem's self-care theory: a tool for education and practice. *Journal of Nursing Education*; **26**(8): 342–3.

Webb C (1986). Introduction: towards a critical analysis of nursing models, in Webb, C. (Ed). *Women's Health, Midwifery and Gynaecological Nursing.* Hodder and Stoughton, London.

Webb N, Hull D and **Madeley R** (1985). Care by parents in hospital. *British Medical Journal*; **291**: 176–7.

9

Caring for a persistent school refuser using a family-centred psychosocial approach
Gillian Chapman

Introduction

Susan was a bright, intelligent 10 year-old who repeatedly refused to go to school, where she had difficulty making friends. Her school work was below standard for her age and ability but her behaviour towards teachers engaging and willing. She was referred to an educational psychologist, where it was discovered that one of the reasons Susan refused to go to school was that she had occasional daytime enuresis. This amounted to occasional moderate to severe wetting of her underwear, of which she was self-conscious. An assessment of organic causes for the enuresis was undertaken at the paediatric unit of the local district general hospital, but physiological functioning was found to be normal. In view of the evident distress these symptoms caused Susan and her family, and the fact that she was failing to meet educational developmental goals, she was referred to a specialist unit able to offer family-centred psychotherapy and a psychosocial approach to the nursing of children and their families. In this chapter an outline of the way in which Susan's problems were assessed and the care plan designed, together with an evaluation and critique of the approach is provided.

First, however, the theoretical and research literature dealing with children with distressing behavioural symptoms is reviewed to put Susan's experience in context.

Review of the literature

There are a range of theoretical models which seek to explain the way psychological distress in children may be expressed in physical symptoms and emotional and behavioural disturbance (Rutter, 1982; Wolf, 1981). Once organic causes for the problems are discounted, the two most compelling explanatory frameworks derive from behavioural psychology (Skinner, 1953; Hall and Lindzey, 1970) and psycho-analytic theory (Stafford-Clarke, 1983). Both models stress the importance of recognizing the disruption to the child's normal development which the symptoms provoke, and both recognize the complexity of the issues involved and the importance of the family in the child's psychopathology. They differ with respect to the stress they place on factors which may cause the disturbance and thus what might be helpful in terms of treatment. For example, a therapist adopting a purely behavioural approach may take the view that maladaptive behaviours (like school refusal) are learnt behaviours. It follows from this that a therapeutic programme designed to modify the behaviour, by using a system of rewards for approved behaviour, would be the treatment of choice. On the other hand, a psychoanalyst would view the behavioural disturbance as a communication about anxieties generated within the family. The treatment of choice would be to explore the child's and family's feelings, thoughts and relationships as a way of generating insight and understanding about the internal conflicts experienced by the child. Psychotherapeutic intervention and interpretation would help the child and parents understand, and therefore overcome or resolve, the sometimes passionate feelings which lead to the distressing behaviour. In practice, of course, many therapists adopt a modified approach based on both disciplines (Brown and Pedder, 1979).

Rutter (1982) points out that most therapeutic approaches adopt the view that childhood disturbance is a more extreme manifestation of ordinary behaviour, and should be understood in terms of the stage of intellectual and psychosocial development the child would ordinarily be expected to have reached. First, he suggests that criteria for assessment of children's problems should include an evaluation of whether the behaviour is abnormal in terms of the child's age and sex, life circumstances and the socio-cultural setting in which it occurs. For example, a three-year-old who had occasional daytime enuresis and displayed clinging behaviour when his mother left him at playschool would not be abnormal! Susan, however, was 10 years old. Second, Rutter suggests that the type of symptom, its frequency, persistence, severity and the extent to which it is a situation specific impairment should be considered together with the extent to which it involves a change in the child's usual behaviour. Finally, Rutter argues that the degree of impairment involved, the suffering, social isolation and interference with normal development and the life of others will affect judgements about therapeutic interventions.

Surveys of normal child health behaviour help clinicians to assess the extent to which the patients' behaviour exists within a normal range. Susan's symptoms of daytime wetting and school refusal can be set in the context of other children's experiences. Tierney and Tierney (1983) point out that potty training and bedwetting, together with temper tantrums and sleep problems, are common problems with which parents cope. They cite Chambers' (1981) study on bedwetting in which daytime and night-time continence was achieved by most children by three years of age. About 25 per cent of children wet the bed at night at 3.5 years, 12.5 per

cent at 5 years, 5 per cent at 10 years and 1 per cent at 15 years old. Using figures like these, Susan's experience of daytime wetting at 10 years is clearly far from ordinary.

Butler and Golding's (1986) survey of a cohort of nearly 14,000 children on their fifth birthday also showed that bedwetting, soiling and daytime wetting were fairly common. For example, 5.4 per cent of the 5 year old boys and 3.0 per cent of the girls in the study soiled their underwear and 8.3 per cent of boys and 12 per cent of girls wet themselves during the day. ('Giggle-wetting' explains the higher percentage of girls!) Bedwetting was associated independently with the number of children in the household, social class and the cultural background of the child. Butler and Golding offer only tentative explanations of their findings and suggest that socio-cultural differences in familial attitudes, communications, and behaviour and stressful life events may delay maturational processes.

Hill (1983) in his review of school refusal cites Hersov and Bergs' (1980) work, which points out that occasional truancy is common. Positive school attendance runs at about 90 per cent. The National Child Development Study showed that 50 per cent of children of 16 years of age occasionally truanted from school. Severe truancy was apparently more rare in 8 per cent of children (Fogelman *et al.*, 1980) while 0.5 per cent of primary school pupils and 20 per cent of secondary school pupils (Galloway, 1976 and 1982) were regularly absent from school. However, Hill (1983) distinguishes between school refusal and truancy. Truancy exists where a child is absent from school without the parents' knowledge or consent. In contrast, school refusal exists where a child is absent from school with the parents' knowledge and to their concern, and in the absence of non-school-linked illness. Alternatively the parents may be withholding their child from school attendance. Hill suggests that causal mechanisms associated with school refusal might include separation anxiety (fear of leaving home or parent), special school-related fears (travel, bullying, elements of the curriculum, etc) and general difficulties in adaptation (low self-esteem, or depression).

From this brief review of the literature, it seems

clear that 10 year old Susan's problem of persistent school refusal and day-time wetting were not only at the extreme edge of the normal range of behaviour, but were also likely to cause social isolation from peers and inhibit her educational development. The therapeutic programme offered to Susan was associated with seeking to understand what lay behind her behaviour in order to ameliorate her situation.

Individual psychotherapy by a child psychotherapist, together with psychosocial, family-centred children's nursing was offered. This approach is explained in the next section.

The psychosocial approach to care

The psychosocial approach to the nursing care of children is informed by psychoanalytic theory, with its stress on the importance of the child's attachment and relationship to the mother as a means of developing a sense of self and capacity for relatedness with others. Brown and Pedder (1979) provide a helpful guide to psychodynamic principles and practice which can only be sketched briefly here. They point out that all psychodynamic therapy derives from the work of Freud (1951). Freud suggested that the tension between the conscious and unconscious mind (where memories and experiences are stored and perhaps 'forgotten') creates the conditions in which the individual's experience and behaviour in the present is influenced (even determined) by past familial experiences. The mind's tripartite structure: the id (pleasurable impulses); the ego (reality-based 'common sense' reasoning); the superego (rewarding and/or punitive internalized parental authority), is created in part out of the conflicts arising from the individual's growth through six developmental stages. The oral stage (0 to 1 year), where total dependence and pleasure associated with sucking gives way to the anal stage (1 to 3 years), where control and production of body products are the focus of the toddler's attention. The phallic/oedipal stage (3 to 5 years) where the child experiences intense

jealousy and desire to possess one parent, gives way to latency, a period of quiescence (5 years to puberty), puberty and adolescence which is followed by adult genitality. It was Freud's notion that difficulties or untoward experiences during these developmental stages were the seat of neurosis and emotional and behavioural problems in adulthood. Often, unresolved conflicts in childhood are returned to and repeated in adult life until the conflict is resolved. Return to earlier developmental stages is called regression; 'forgetting' earlier experiences is called repression or denial. The psychoanalyst's job is to be attentive to the patient's accounts of his/her feelings and, via interpretation, render unconscious/repressed material available to the patient's consciousness. It is the experience of being understood, and of understanding early experience, which releases the patient's energy (libido) for more creative, healthy activities.

Freud's daughter, Anna Freud (1966), took these ideas developed in the treatment of adult patients, and applied them to the treatment of disturbed children.

Melanie Klein (1963), later revised Freud's ideas about the key developmental stages, stressing early oral experience as the means by which the child learned about 'good and bad' mothering. Bowlby (1968, 1969, 1980) examined the importance of attachment and loss in emotional and behavioural disturbance. Winnicott's idea of the 'good enough' mother (Phillips, 1988), who provides the environment in which the infant can play, experiment, and test out the strength of the mother's commitment, informs psychosocial nursing most directly. The complexities of adopting this approach are documented in Barnes (1968) and Kennedy *et al.* (1987) and it will not be possible to explore these issues in detail here. Basically, the nurse acknowledges the importance of the mother/parents; not only to the child as a figure of attachment from whom separation would be painful, but also in the creation of the child's disturbance and the capacity of the therapeutic team to resolve this disturbance. In short, a child's emotional and behavioural disturbance is seen as a function and reflection of troubles within the family rather than an isolated symptom.

However, before developing the discussion of care further, it is worth noting that experimental psychologists dismiss Freud's postulation of the tripartite structure of the mind. Experimental psychologists claim that Freud's conceptualization of the mind is not supported by empirical evidence. The psychosocial approach is, therefore, seated in psychoanalytical theory rather than experimental psychology.

Psychosocial nursing seeks, therefore, to understand the psychodynamics of family life while planning and implementing practical care around the ordinary activities of daily living (Roper *et al.*, 1980, 1983; Chapman, 1984) in the context of supportive and perceptive counselling. It is in recognition of the importance of working through difficulties in relationships that one primary nurse is allocated to care for the family throughout their stay in the unit. The nurse works in partnership with the family and psychotherapist, who share a responsibility for treatment and for using the associate nurse in the primary nurse's absence. Primary nursing is used, not as an organizational or managerial exercise, but precisely because it facilitates the development of a trusting relationship with the family, out of which understanding and insight into family dynamics is developed. The psychoanalytic concept of transference and counter-transference is used to understand the relationship which develops between the nurse and family. The nurse, together with the therapist, reflects upon the way she feels about and responds to members of the family. Fairly commonly, one or more members of the family may act towards the nurse as if she or he were a parental figure (Macklin, 1979). For example, Susan's mother, Mrs Jones, either responded to the nurse in a contemptuous and rejecting way, or overwhelmed her with over solicitous enquiries about her health. At the same time, Mrs Jones idealized the psychotherapist, perceiving him as being both caring and clever. As will become clearer later in the case history, these responses were reminiscent of Mrs Jones's characteristic way of responding to her own mother (whom she considered was cold and timid) and father (whom she considered was warm but domineering). It will later be shown that discussions between the therapist, nurse and patient about transference and counter-transference issues of this type, helped Mrs Jones to develop insight into not only her own behaviour, but her daughter's dilemma. The therapeutic programme available to Mrs Jones and her daughter Susan is outlined in Figure 9.1.

There are five elements worthy of note. Firstly, the use of the therapeutic community and ordinary everyday activities as a therapeutic tool – no drugs were included in the treatment. Secondly, the

OPD: Initial interview with doctor and primary nurse to assess history and suitability for treatment.

Home visit: To observe family relationships in natural setting, identify problems associated with admission, and act as a bridge between home and unit.

Pre-admission/admission: To facilitate reception of family into unit, and observe initial reactions.

Assessment review: To observe, assess and evaluate the family's ability to use therapeutic community/programme.

Triage review: Multidisciplinary meeting to use observations of family to deepen understanding of problems and formulate care plans.

Regular review: To consider development and progress.

Discharge planning: To facilitate discharge of family home.

Figure 9.1 The assessment process.

importance of nursing in the transition from home to hospital expressed in a domiciliary visit before admission. Other writers (Robertson, 1970; Jolly, 1981; Hawthorne, 1974; Fradd, 1986), concerned with the care of children in hospital have stressed the importance of preparing children for admission, and of involving parents and significant others in the care. Thirdly, the importance of regular review meetings in which the progress of the family and staff's responses to them are discussed. Staff support systems of this kind are essential where the quality of work is psychologically intensive. Fourthly, the contract with the family which stresses their joint responsibility in ensuring the integrity of the therapeutic programme. Finally, the importance of providing a safe environment in which feelings may be expressed and disagreements aired without precipitate action being taken or permanent harm created. The nursing care plan together with a brief history of Susan's difficulties are provided in Figures 9.2 a–f.

Evaluating the approach to care

Reconstructing a care plan in the format demanded of a chapter imposes a misleading order and coherence to the nursing care provided. In psychotherapeutic work presenting problems may be known at the beginning of the therapeutic encounter and hypotheses generated about underlying psycho-dynamic factors, but the specific goal of the therapeutic journey is largely unknown. It is therefore difficult to evaluate and measure the outcomes of interventions. This is because the patient's development of understanding about how and why they feel and act as they do is very much a process of discovery. Thus nursing care plans are required which are flexible enough to accommodate the emergent and unexpected responses of the family to the therapeutic process. This makes planning outcomes in terms of precise and measurable behaviour somewhat uncertain. For example, during the period of caring for Susan, the therapeutic team recognized and attended to her mother's difficulties with relationships and collusion with Susan's school refusal. Mrs Jones discovered for herself during her therapy how depressed, angry and disappointed she had felt during her own childhood about her parent's lack of acknowledgement of her academic potential at school. Her father had refused to support her at university. Mrs Jones felt that although her father was a loving and passionate man, he was also controlling and dominating. Her mother, she felt, lacked warmth and seemed passive and timid in contrast. It became clearer to Mrs Jones that her marriage and current intimate relationship with a neighbour, Peter, re-enacted elements of this learned conjugal dynamic behaviour. She saw how Susan, by refusing to go to school and by expressing her feelings silently by wetting during the day, was in some way acting out and attempting to compensate for her mother's disappointment.

Winnicott (1958; 1964; 1984) provides theoretical insight into the difficulties children with depressed parents (such as Susan) might encounter. Phillips (1988) cites Winnicott: 'A child with a depressed mother could . . . feel infinitely dropped' (p.30). Such a child must first seek to deal with the mother's mood and care for her in the (impossible) hope that she will eventually establish the mother she needs to facilitate her own growth. One way of doing this may be to identify with and take on the mother's depression, seeking to cheer her up. By doing this the child sacrifices her own primary wish to be understood and is distracted from her own developmental goals. A depressed mother may, in short, reverse the process where she provides an environment in which the child may grow, by using the child to sustain something in herself.

In Mrs Jones's case, her attempts to provide Susan with the love she felt she had not received had led to her colluding with Susan's clinging behaviour when separation was imminent. It was out of this discovery that Mrs Jones began to think about her relationship with Peter, and managing his domineering relationship with Susan. The family's primary nurse responded to this wish by arranging and attending a family meeting with Mrs Jones, Peter and Susan, where some of these issues were discussed, and the ground rules of the relationships were renegotiated.

It became clear that the issue of schooling had

Aim	Observations	Intervention	Evaluation
To obtain history of current problem	10-year-old Susan lives alone with her mother. Bright intelligent child of first marriage. Visits father who now has new wife and children. School refusal and enuresis for last two years. Very attached to mother who had 'nervous' trouble following divorce. Mother now has an intimate relationship with Peter – a neighbour – who sought to act as a proxy father to Susan.	Attempt to establish rapport.	Mrs Jones able to talk about the difficulties and collaborate over the date of the home visit. Given precise directions etc.
To identify parent's perception of the problem.	Mrs Jones believes Susan is hurt by her father's remarriage two years ago.	Attentive listening and non-judgemental attitude.	
To identify the child's perception of the problem.	Susan 'likes the teachers' but thinks school is 'horrible'.		
To assess capacity to use psycho-social approach.	Susan's enuresis and school refusal suggest regression to prior happier stage of development. Separation anxiety. Mother has some capacity for insight.	Arrange a date for home visit.	

Figure 9.2a First interview.

Aim	Observation/Assessment	Intervention	Evaluation
To make initial assessment of family in own environment.	Home is a 2-bedroomed council flat – scrupulously clean and tidy. Mrs Jones welcoming but anxious. Peter called in during visit and scolded Susan for giving her mother trouble. Mrs Jones accepted this.	Observation of family dynamics.	Peter/Susan dynamic observed together with mother's passivity when Susan was scolded. Checked if arrangements understood.
To identify admission difficulties.	Mother has part-time job. Susan said she'd miss her budgerigar.	Provided information re travel arrangements to mothers job, and supported decision to keep it. Suggested Peter looked after the budgerigar – agreed. Weekend trips home encouraged.	
To facilitate transition from home to hospital.	Mrs Jones and Susan asked many questions about hospital life, what to bring, etc.	Information given.	Mrs Jones and Susan arrived at the time and date arranged.

Figure 9.2b Home visit.

Aim	Observation/Assessment	Intervention	Evaluation
To prepare environment and other patients.	Mrs Jones and Susan very anxious on arrival.	Other patients invited to choose room and select a patient 'mentor'. Nurse checks room, laundry facilities, school placement.	Mrs Jones and Susan settled in talking with other patients. Content with room. Mrs Jones understands therapeutic programme. Susan attended school on the first day but cried piteously when her mother tried to leave her.
To receive family and to receive initial reactions.	Other patients supportive.	Mrs Jones and Susan informed about programme and introduced to patient 'mentor'.	

Figure 9.2c Pre-admission/admission.

Aim	Observation/Assessment	Intervention	Evaluation
To discuss with multidisciplinary team assessment of problems and formulate plans for future treatment and nursing care.	The school refusal is conceptualized as a function of Susan's separation anxiety following the breakup of her mother's marriage to her father and his subsequent new family. It was suggested that Susan felt unable to leave her mother in case she (Mrs Jones) became seriously depressed and left her. The daytime enuresis seems to occur when she is angry or upset about her school work. Mrs Jones's inability to be firm with Susan is seen as a function of her own guilt about the marriage breakdown and underlying depression about her own parents.	Involve Susan in hospital activities with other children to develop social skills.	Susan occasionally spontaneously involved in play activities with other children.
		Facilitate Susan's attendance at school, tailing off her mother as an escort, and encourage Susan to go with her friends.	Attends school by herself.
	Susan's reading age was about 8.4 years on the NEALE analysis of reading ability and comprehension. At school she was beginning to make friends with peers, risking the teacher's disapproval from time to time. Susan was beginning to explore her feelings with the child psychotherapist and making good use of the play materials.	Help mother think through pleasant activities she, Susan and Peter could share, and arrange regular weekend trips home.	Weekends at home fairly enjoyable although arguments do arise.
		Continue personal hygiene routine.	
	In Mrs Jones's psychotherapy early feelings about her family background and disappointment began to emerge in the context of her current relationship with Peter. Both Mrs Jones and Susan appeared to be making good use of the therapeutic programme.	Offer Mrs Jones regular meeting time to support her through her depression.	Mrs Jones becoming increasingly depressed/Peter wants them to leave hospital.

Figure 9.2d Initial assessment.

Aim	Observation/Assessment	Intervention	Evaluation
To observe mother/daughter relationship.	Mrs Jones and Susan appear very attached to each other. Susan is clinging when her mother leaves for work or when she has to go to school. Mrs Jones seems to lack the ability to be firm, and dithers between staying and leaving until she loses her temper and separates violently.	Be available to Mrs Jones and Susan at times of separation, acknowledge feelings, but be firm regarding school attendance, etc. Suggest alternative ways they can be together (eg. cooking etc.).	Number and quality of separation episodes recorded and activities formulated which make separation easier.
To assess extent of enuresis, timing and frequency.	Susan's enuretic episodes are confined to occasional wetting at school and night-time enuresis since admission.	Encourage Mrs Jones to involve Susan in her own laundry. Agree a regular post-meal toilet regime with Susan and her mother. Use gold star and chart system.	Progress monitored on chart.
To observe Susan's school attendance.	Susan enjoys maths and reading at school but will only attend if her mother escorts her. There are frequently emotional scenes as she says goodbye.	Arrange for Susan to go to school with another pupil and her parents.	School attendance checked with teacher, Susan and mother.
To observe Mrs Jones' and Susan's use of the therapeutic programme.	Mrs Jones and Susan both make use of the therapeutic programme offered – taking the opportunity to speak in meetings.	Agree regular 'counselling' sessions to explore feelings, etc.	Reflect on 'counselling' material and discuss as appropriate with multidisciplinary team.

Figure 9.2e Continuing assessment.

Aim	Observation/Assessment	Intervention	Evaluation
To identify residual difficulties.	Susan's difficulties have largely resolved but Mrs Jones remains depressed.	Liaise with school authorities and educational psychologist and school nurse about Susan's return to school.	Mrs Jones and Susan left hospital sad but relatively content about discharge arrangements. Mrs Jones regularly attends OPD and reports that Susan only rarely refuses to go to school. The daytime enuresis has ceased.
To facilitate the transition from hospital to home.	Mrs Jones and Susan both anxious about leaving hospital in case problems return. Both are sad about leaving relationships developed with patients and staff.	Acknowledge feelings of loss.	
To arrange suitable long term support for the family.	Mrs Jones requires further out-patient psychotherapy.	Arrange out-patient psychotherapy for Mrs Jones. Inform GP about treatment and progress.	

Figure 9.2f Discharge planning.

become a battleground for Susan. On the one hand her unconscious wish was to keep her mother constantly in sight to protect against further losses, on the other, was a wish to express her own autonomy against Peter's domineering attitude to her school attendance. (See the domiciliary visit report.) Together, Peter and Mrs Jones acknowledged that they needed to work on the uncertainties in their own relationship and the extent of their commitment to each other, rather than concentrating their joint attention on Susan's behavioural difficulties. Furthermore, it became clear that although Susan's natural father had not wished to be involved in the therapeutic programme, he did want to maintain and develop his relationship with her, retaining the paternal role in which Peter was so inadequate. To this end, the nurses helped Mrs Jones to plan and cope with Susan's sometimes painful weekends in her father's new household.

As Susan's mother acknowledged her own depression and focused her attention on her own difficult relationships, Susan was to some extent released from her role as the family problem. She grew more confident in her ability to make friends at school and her daytime enuresis came under control. Indeed, she began to become impatient with the limitations of the hospital school and expressed an interest in returning to her own school at home.

This extended example of the way growing insight within the family may help resolve childrens' distress, demonstrates how important flexibility is in planning care in psychosocial nursing. It is this flexibility, determined by the emergent nature of psychological growth, which makes measuring the outcome of nursing care uncertain.

Difficulties in predicting and measuring the outcome of psychosocial nursing are shared by psychotherapeutic work generally. At a formal level Eysenck and Wilson (1973) claim that psychoanalytic theory cannot be substantiated empirically. Kline (1982) discusses why this might be true in his summary of the conclusions of research evaluating psychoanalytic theory and practice. Firstly, research studies evaluating psychotherapeutic treatment assume that patients are a homogeneous group, rarely include enough therapists to ensure statistical validity, and have no fixed, generally agreed criteria for successful therapeutic outcomes. Secondly, in the field of psychiatry generally, it is difficult to establish whether the patient would have recovered spontaneously.

Feminist theorists have criticized psychoanalytic theory, not only for its lack of insight into the psychology of women, but the way culture determines their life chances and opportunities (Mitchell, 1975; Eichenbaum and Orbach, 1985). It has been suggested that these failings distort the nature of psychotherapeutic work undertaken with women.

At a more practical level, most practitioners consider that patients suffering from the neuroses do better than those with psychotic illnesses. The capacity for insight, self-responsibility and the ability to talk through problems rather than act them out, together with a willingness to develop a therapeutic alliance with the therapist, are also pre-requisites to successful therapy. While the criticism that some patients and their families lack psychological sophistication and insight and cannot benefit from the therapeutic approach may be accurate, it does not follow from this, as some critics have suggested, that only middle class articulate families can benefit. What matters is the patient's capacity to distinguish between his or her feelings and those of others, and to own responsibility for his or her own behaviour and responses to others (Chapman, 1990).

Another practical problem associated with adopting the principles of psychosocial nursing and psychoanalytic theory is that the full psychotherapeutic programme described here requires specialist skills not always available in every locality. Furthermore, not all families are able or willing to commit the time and energy required. In Susan's case the admission lasted about seven months. The experience is intensive for the staff team as well as the family, and adequate support systems, clinical supervision and training are required. The strength of the psychosocial approach, for those able to use it and where the facilities are available, lies in the respect it offers the family and child, and the primacy of their feelings in determining behaviour and experiences. Psychoanalytically inspired psychosocial nursing, like good mothering, provides the psychological and social context in which child and family feel safe enough to test out their feelings and have the experience of being understood.

Acknowledgements

The views and errors found in this chapter are, of course, those of the author but I am grateful to Mrs Daphne Patey, Principal Nursing Officer, Department of Health, for her thoughtful reading of the text.

References

Barnes E (1968). *Psychosocial Nursing*. Tavistock Publications, London.

Berg I (1985). The management of truancy. *Journal of Child Psychological Psychiatry*; **26(3)**: 325–31.

Bowlby J (1968). *Attachment and Loss: I Attachment*. Hogarth Press, London.

Bowlby J (1969). *Attachment and Loss: II Separation, Anxiety and Anger*. Hogarth Press, London.

Bowlby J (1980). *Attachment and Loss: III Loss, Sadness and Depression*. Basic Books, New York.

Brown D and Pedder J (1979). *Introduction to Psychotherapy. An Outline of Psychodynamic Principles and Practice*. Tavistock Publications, London and New York.

Butler N and Golding J (1986). *From Birth to Five*. Pergamon Press, Oxford.

Chambers T (1981). Fears and tears. *Nursing Mirror*; **153(24)**: 52–3.

Chapman GE (1984). A therapeutic community, psychosocial nursing and the nursing process. *International Journal of Therapeutic Communities*; **5(2)**: 1984.

Chapman GE (1990). Individual psychotherapy and counselling, in Brooking J (Ed), *A Textbook in Psychiatric Nursing* (In press).

Eichenbaum L and Orbach S (1985). *Understanding Women*. Penguin Books, Harmondsworth, Middlesex.

Eysenck HJ and Wilson GD (1973). *The Experimental Study of Freudian Theory*. Methuen, London and New York.

Fogelman K, Tibbeham A and Lambert L (1980). Out of School, in Hersov L and Bergs I (Eds) *Out of School; Modern Perspectives in Truancy and School Refusal*, John Wiley, Chichester.

Fradd E (1986). Learning about hospital. *Nursing Times*; **15 Jan**: 28–30.

Freud A (1966). *Normality and Pathology in Childhood*. Hogarth Press, London.

Freud S (1951). *Complete Psychological Works*. Hogarth Press, London.

Galloway D (1976). Persistent unjustified absence from school. *Trends in Education*; **4**: 22–7.

Galloway D (1982). Persistent absence from school. *Educational Research*; **24(3)**: 188–96.

Hall CS and Lindzey G (1970). *Theories of Personality*, 2nd Edition, John Wiley, Chichester.

Hawthorne PJ (1974). *Nurse, I Want My Mummy*. Royal College of Nursing, London.

Hersov L and Bergs I (eds) (1980). *Out of School: Modern Perspectives in Truancy and School Refusal*. John Wiley, Chichester.

Hill P (1983). Children who refuse to go to school. Parts 1 and 2. *Maternal and Child Health*; **Feb–Mar**: 118–20.

Jolly J (1981). *The Other Side of Paediatrics*. Macmillan, London.

Kennedy R, Heyman A and Tischler L (1987). *The Family as Inpatient*. Free Association Press, London.

Klein M (1963). *The Psychoanalysis of Children*. Hogarth Press, London.

Kline P (1982). *Fact and Fantasy in Freudian Theory*. Methuen, London and New York.

Macklin D (1979). Trouble stirring in the kitchen. *Nursing Mirror*; **May 24**: 38–9.

Mitchell J (1975). *Psychoanalysis and Feminism*. Penguin Books, Harmondsworth, Middlesex.

Phillips A (1988). *Winnicott*. Fontana Modern Masters. F. Kermode (ed), Fontana Press, Glasgow. pp. 30.

Robertson J (1970). *Young Children in Hospital*. 2nd Edition, Tavistock Publications, Cambridge.

Roper N, Logan W and Tierney A (1980). *The Elements of Nursing*. Churchill Livingstone, London.

Roper N, Logan W and Tierney A (1983). *Using a Model of Nursing*. Churchill Livingstone, London.

Rutter M (1982). *Helping Troubled Children*. Penguin Books, Harmondsworth, Middlesex.

Skinner BF (1953). *Science and Human Behaviour*. Macmillan, New York.

Stafford-Clarke D (1983). *What Freud Really Said*. Penguin Books, Harmondsworth, Middlesex.

Tierney A and Tierney I (1983). Perennial problems of parenthood. *Nursing*; **19**: 546–51.

Winnicott DW (1958). *Collected Papers; Through Paediatrics to Psychoanalysis*. Tavistock, London.

Winnicott DW (1964). *The Family and Individual Development*. Tavistock, London.

Winnicott DW (1984). *The Child, the Family and the Outside World*. Penguin Books, Harmondsworth, Middlesex.

Wolf S (1981). *Children Under Stress*. 2nd Edition, Penguin Books, Harmondsworth, Middlesex.

10

Health teaching in a primary school using Becker's health belief model

Alison While

Introduction

Children spend at least 11 years at school during their childhood years and therefore experiences in school life play an important part in the development of the future adult. This chapter attempts to demonstrate how the educational potential of school nursing may be developed using a health belief model (Becker *et al.*, 1974) to guide practice. The subject matter of the health teaching was reflective of current parental concerns. However, it is not suggested that education pertaining to AIDS is the only worthwhile topic.

The school health service

The need for a school health service was recognized in the late nineteenth century, and the urgency for its existence was further highlighted by the poor physical condition of Boer War army recruits (Interdepartmental Committee, 1904). Much has changed since those early days, however, but the aim of the school health service continues to be to ensure that children are physically and emotionally healthy so that they may benefit fully from their education and thereby achieve their full potential, and prepare them for parenthood and ensure their optimum health in adult life (Carpenter, 1985). Indeed, Carpenter has asserted:

'For eleven years of their lives, all children are in contact with this service which has the potential to affect them significantly.'

(p.1167)

Research examining the role of the school nurse within the school health service is very limited and the only major published survey was carried out in 1973 (Thurmott, 1976). Whilst acknowledging that much has changed regarding all aspects of health care provision since 1973, the findings of this survey describe the continuing elements of school nursing practice, namely the routine screening and surveillance of the school population, the selection of children for and preparation of school medical medical examinations, the follow-up of 'vulnerable' school children, counselling and health education. Indeed, both Shannon (1984) and Hawes (1989) in describing their role acknowledge involvement in all these areas of work.

The Court Report (DHSS, 1976) was the first enquiry to critically examine the provision of health care for school children since the inception of the National Health Service. Among many other recommendations, this report stressed the need for strengthening the school health service with an improved nursing provision so that the school nurse could function effectively as 'the representative of health in the everyday life of the school' (para. 10.13).

Indeed, the report argued that this important contribution was frequently overlooked and undervalued. The report further stated that the school nurse:

'... has a special contribution to make in the curriculum planning and provision of health education in the school, and in individual health teaching and counselling of pupils.'

(para 10.13)

However, despite the immense potential of the school health service there is evidence that it is failing to meet the needs of the population it serves and that the quality of the service is variable (National Childrens Bureau – NCB, 1987; Hall, 1989; While, 1989a). Further, the school health service has restricted its performance to routine screening rather than interpreting its role in a broader sense as an agent of health education and promotion within the educational setting.

AIDS as a potential health problem

An outbreak of opportunist diseases was first observed among previously healthy homosexual men in the United States during 1981 (McEvoy, 1987). The evidence suggested that the syndrome was caused by a blood-borne and sexually transmissible virus which was isolated in 1983 by Martagnier and Gallo. It is now known as human immunodeficiency virus (HIV).

Epidemiological evidence suggests that heterosexual spread is common in Africa and is occurring in Europe and the United States, although its spread in the United Kingdom appears to be at a relatively early stage. In the Mediterranean countries the fastest growing outbreak is among intravenous drug abusers, many of whom are women of child-bearing age (McEnvoy, 1987). Pinching (1986) has argued that we must learn lessons from the African epidemic in which the issue of AIDS has been clouded by misinformation, ignorance, rumour and uninformed speculation.

There is evidence that the level of public knowledge is limited which perhaps reflects the coverage of the issue in the national press. Currie

(1987) found that the popular newspapers were considerably less educational than the quality press regarding information about how to protect oneself from contracting the virus. Indeed, he viewed their coverage at best useless and at worst worrying and designed solely for entertainment. However, since there is no available effective therapy or vaccination at present, the only means of tackling the pandemic rests upon primary prevention founded on wide-reaching public health campaigns highlighting essential information.

The future of a nation rests upon its school children for they are the parents of tomorrow. Further, 'healthy' habits are established during the early years of life (While, 1989b). And it is also inevitable that some HIV infected children (perinatal infected and haemophiliacs) will be attending schools (Bloom, 1988) and they deserve humane treatment by their peers. An educational programme therefore clearly has a place in a sound school health service provision if inaccurate and incomplete knowledge is to be remedied (Chief Medical Officer, 1986).

The health education model

The health belief model (Becker *et al.*, 1974) drew heavily upon the work of Kurt Lewin (1935). The model has a phenomenological orientation and assumes that the subjective world of the perceiver rather than the objective environment determines behaviour (Rosenstock, 1966). Accordingly, it is proposed that the likelihood that a person will take action regarding a disease is determined both by the individual's psychological state of readiness to take action and by the perceived benefit of action weighed against the perceived cost or barriers involved in the proposed action. The individual's psychological state of readiness to action is determined by both perceived susceptibility to the particular disease and the perceived severity of the consequences of contracting the disease. Thus action will not occur unless the individual believes in both personal susceptibility and the seriousness of the disease, should it occur. (See Figure 7.1 p. 63.)

There is sufficient wealth of research to support the empirical adequacy of the health belief model (e.g. McKinlay, 1972; Becker *et al.*, 1974; Mikhail, 1981, Gatchel and Baum, 1983; Champion, 1984; While, 1986). Further, the model gives insight into why people behave in certain ways regarding their health and what factors may affect their decision-making process. The model suggests that both demographic and sociopsychological variables play their part in formulating behaviour, along with structural variables which includes knowledge base and cues to action. However, the model implicitly assumes that the individual person is the ultimate unit of analysis and that a generalization can be made from a study of individual behaviour. This may not be possible. The model has also been criticized for not explaining the nature and form of the influence of modifying variables upon the individual's perceptions and beliefs and how these are expressed in resultant behaviour. However, neither Rosenstock and Kirscht (1974) nor Haefner (1974) claimed the model to be complete but rather argued that it provided a scientific foundation for the understanding of health behaviour, and in so doing suggested a number of potential strategies for changing health behaviour. The model suggests that direct persuasion as well as other strategies may prove effective – the removal of barriers to action may also produce the desired outcome. In the circumstances of this chapter when clearly children are developing their beliefs and behaviour, the emphasis will be placed upon improving their knowledge base and that of their families.

Assessment of a primary school class

Mrs. B's class consists of 30 pupils all of whom have either had their sixth birthday or will be six within the next few months. There are 13 boys and 17 girls of mixed ethnic backgrounds with both Asians and West Indians well represented. No class member is known to be HIV infected although one school pupil is a haemophiliac. One third of the children are from single parent households and most families would be categorized as coming from the social classes III, IV and V using the Registrar General's classification.

The knowledge of the group is very limited regarding how their bodies work and questions about AIDS elicit laughter followed by grossly inaccurate knowledge.

The context of health teaching

The health belief model (Becker *et al.*, 1974) highlights the context within which individuals take decisions regarding the adoption of a health life-style. Among the 'modifying factors', the model includes demographic and sociopsychological variables and therefore explicitly acknowledges the influence of parents and teachers upon the decision making process. Knowledge of the subject matter is considered to be a structural variable which also play its part in the assessment of the worth of a particular health action.

Effective health education among young school children will therefore depend upon the preparation of class teachers and parents, who will not only act as role models, but also act as a source of information when the children seek explanations for their concerns arising from any formal teaching. Although the school nurse has a continuing presence in the school, access to her is limited to the occasions when she is carrying out duties within the school. Prior to the formal teaching sessions with the children, the parents and teachers were therefore provided with supporting literature and invited to two separate briefing sessions – the parent session was held at 6pm on a weekday and the teacher session was held during a lunch break.

While this chapter emphasizes AIDS education, the topic was not addressed in isolation but was part of a continuing health education programme. Indeed, it was one of a number of topics generated during a parent's 'health' evening at the school. The school facilitates health education by allocating one large noticeboard in a prominent place for the staging of poster and literature displays to develop the health themes under consideration within the school. The school nurse encourages consultation and discussions during her scheduled school attendance for advisory and health surveillance purposes.

The teaching plan

School curriculum time is very restricted especially with the introduction of the National Curriculum. The teaching plan was therefore organized over two forty-minute sessions. The children were given supporting literature to take home to discuss with their parents.

Lesson I – Addressing children's knowledge deficit

Aims
- Give a general overview of how the body protects itself from infections.
- Describe the meaning of the terms 'germs' and 'viruses'.
- Interest the group in the subject.

Learning outcomes
- Develop a limited understanding of the function of the skin and the immune system.
- Gain some understanding of 'germ' and 'virus' and how they are transmitted.

Strategy
- Discuss who has had a recent cold – why? How did they get it? Why do we blow our noses? . . .
- Talk about the experience of having an injection – what happens to the needle hole? . . .
- Ask the children to draw a leg with a new cut/graze on the knee and then ask them to redraw the same leg when the cut/graze has healed up – discuss these drawings.

Assessment strategy
- Rapport and discussion with the group.
- Discussion with individual pupils when undertaking routine health surveillance work.
- Feedback from class teacher and parents both during informal and formal contact e.g. parents' health evening.

Lesson II – Addressing children's knowledge deficit and providing advice regarding a healthy lifestyle

Aims
- Introduce the topic of AIDS.
- Explore group's knowledge and correct inaccuracies.
- Reduce amount of misinformation.

Learning outcomes
- Develop an introductory understanding of AIDS and how the disease is spread within the context of a child's life.
- A realistic anxiety about AIDS.

Strategy
- Discuss what they know about AIDS – correct inaccurate knowledge particularly regarding modes of transmission.
- Discuss good hygiene habits for own well-being e.g. washing hands, not engaging in blood brother and sister games.
- Ask the children to draw themselves and then ask them to draw a child of the same age with AIDS – discuss these drawings.

Assessment strategy
- Rapport and discussion with group.
- Discussion with individual pupils when undertaking routine health surveillance work.
- Feedback from class teacher and parents both during informal and formal contact.

The future

Changes in school education with the introduction of the National Curriculum means that health education is part of the educational programme. The school nurse has the potential to become the prime source of information and facilitator of health promotion within the school. With the realization of this potential, school leavers should in future be able to reap the benefits of making sound informed decisions regarding their health, lifestyle and relationships. AIDS education will be but a part of this role. The benefits of health education among children are now well accepted for it seems that the primary socialization phase, when attitudes and value systems are created, is the most receptive educational phase. Attempts at modifying well-established values and behaviour in later life are considerably more difficult.

The health belief model (Becker *et al.*, 1974) provides a useful framework upon which to base health teaching and permits an understanding of the difficult area of health beliefs and health behaviour.

However, the inducing of high perceived severity through education may be ineffective in producing appropriate health behaviour unless accompanied by instructions about how to cope with the threat or reduce the danger (Krishner *et al.*, 1973). Without a recommended way to reduce the danger, individuals use denial as a defence mechanism to restore emotional balance. This linear relationship between fear arousal and action is referred to as the Yorkes-Dodson effect (Tones, 1977) and highlights the necessity of providing advice about healthy lifestyles. Indeed, research in psychology increasingly endorses the importance of perceived benefits and barriers to action as determinants of health behaviour (Gatchel and Baum, 1983). Therefore advice should permit individuals to find the adoption of a healthy lifestyle an easy choice and in the context of this chapter, the adoption of good hygiene habits should be demonstrated as not only wise but involving no great inconvenience to the child.

The British research literature demonstrates a wealth of work in health education ranging from large studies to small projects which form the majority. However, most of the research has no explicit theoretical base and as such does not address itself to the study of interactions between health beliefs and consequent health behaviour. Furthermore, like much of the American research, modifying variables have not been tested independently so it is difficult to draw any conclusions. Interestingly, Kasl (1974) has argued that the variables are independent and this was supported by Champion's (1984) research. But Redman (1980) has doubted the total indpendence of the variables and suggested that the variables could be interrelated or cumulatively interrelated. More research addressing this area is clearly needed.

The health belief model of Becker *et al.* (1974) however, highlights the importance of individual perceptions and the role of modifying factors in the decision-making process of selecting the mode of behaviour. The uncertainty about the spread of AIDS within the United Kingdom makes it imperative that school children are given every opportunity to develop an understanding of the problem and how they may avoid acquiring it in the future. It has been argued that the school nurse has the potential to make a major contribution to the well being of the next generation of adults through the provision of information and facilitation based upon the health belief model.

References

Becker MH, Drachman RH and **Kirscht JP** (1974). A new approach to explaining sick role behaviour in low income populations. *American Journal of Public Health*; **64**: 205–16.

Bloom AL (1988). Acquired immune deficiency syndrome in childhood. *Public Health*; **102**: 97–106.

Carpenter MJ (1985). *Health Care of the School Child*. Bailliere Tindall, London.

Champion VL (1984). Instrument development for health belief model constructs. *Advances in Nursing Science*; **6(3)**: 73–85.

Chief Medical Officer (1986). Children at school and problems related to AIDS. Letter. *CMO*; **(86)1**. DHSS, London.

Currie CE (1987). *Press Health Coverage in UK National, Scottish National and Scottish Local Press*. Research Unit in Health and Behavioural Change, University of Edinburgh.

DHSS (1976). *Fit for the Future*. Report of the Committee on Child Health Services Cmnd 6684. Vol. 1. Chairman: Professor SDM Court, HMSO, London.

Gatchel RJ and **Baum A** (1983). *An Introduction to Health Psychology*. Addison-Wesley, Reading, Mass., USA.

Haefner D (1974). The health relief model and preventive dental behaviour. *Health Education Monograph*; **2(4)**: 420–32.

Hall DMB (1989). *Health for All Children*. Oxford Medical, Oxford.

Hawes M (1989). School nursing in Norwich Health Authority. *Health Visitor*; **62(11)**: 351–2.

Interdepartmental Committee (1904). *Report of the Interdepartmental Committee on Physical Deterioration*. Cmnd 2175. Vol. 1. HMSO, London.

Kasl SV (1974). The health belief model and behaviour related to chronic illness. *Health Education Monograph*; **2(4)**: 420–5.

Krisher HP, Darley SA and **Darley JM** (1973). Fear provoking recommendations; intentions to take preventive actions and actual preventive actions. *Journal of Personality and Social Psychology*; **26(2)**: 301–8.

Lewin K (1935). *A Dynamic Theory of Personality*. McGraw-Hill, New York.

McEvoy M (1987). The epidemiology of AIDS. *Institute of Medical Ethics Bulletin*; **Supplement 4**: 3.

McKinlay JB (1972). Some approaches and problems in the study of the uses of services – an overview. *Journal of Health and Social Behaviour*, **13(2)**: 115–52.

Mikhail B (1981). The health belief model: a review and critical evaluation of the model, research and practice. *Advances of Nursing Science*, **4(1)**: 65–82.

National Children's Bureau (1987). *Investing in the Future: Child Health Ten Years After the Court Report*. NCB, London.

Pinching AJ (1986). AIDS and Africa: lessons for us all. *Journal of Royal Society of Medicine*; **79**: 501–3.

Redman BK (1980). *The Process of Patient Teaching in Nursing*. CV Mosby, St Louis.

Rosenstock IM (1966). Why people use health services. *Milbank Memorial Fund Quarterly*; **44(1)**: 94–123.

Rosenstock IM and Kirscht JP (1974). Practice implications. *Health Education Monograph*; **2(4)**: 328–35.

Shannon A (1984). Exeter's new concept of the school nurse Role. *Health Visitor*, **57(5)**: 150–1.

Thurmott P (1976). *Health and the School*. Royal College of Nursing, London.

Tones BK (1977). *Effectiveness and efficiency in health education: a review of theory and practice*. Occasional Paper. Scottish Health Education Unit, Edinburgh.

While AE (1986). The uptake of prophylactic care during infancy, in While AE (ed), *Research in Preventive Community Nursing Care*. John Wiley, Chichester.

While AE (1989a). *The Health Experience of Primary School Children*. Unpublished Report.

While AE (1989b). *Health in the Inner City*. Heinemann Medical, Oxford.

11

Caring for an adolescent girl with anorexia nervosa using Cawley's levels of psychotherapy
Susan Ritter

Adolescence

Adolescence marks a transitional stage between childhood and adulthood which may be relatively trouble-free, but in groups seen by mental health professionals adolescence is often very troubled, ranging from the 'seriously impaired' to the 'sensitive and vulnerable' (King, 1972, p.364). The maturational changes of adolescence occur and are 'regulated by a generically determined time schedule' which is 'relatively independent of environmental events'. But physical and psychological maturation can be disrupted by environmental events that are extreme enough (Atkinson *et al.*, 1987).

Anorexia nervosa has the effect of preventing or reversing maturational processes (Figure 11.1).

- emaciation
- poor peripheral circulation
- bradycardia
- postural hypotension
- low mood
- amenorrhoea
- intolerance of cold
- impotence
- ± oedema
- ↓ basal metabolic rate
- ↓ body temperature
- preoccupation with food
- characterization of self as fat

Figure 11.1 Clinical features of anorexia nervosa.

The weight loss can obscure the development of secondary sexual characteristics, and eventually disrupts endocrinological functions enough to cause amenorrhoea. However, weight loss does not itself delay the appearance of secondary sexual characteristics, and amenorrhoea may precede as well as follow weight loss in emaciated young women, making the causal link difficult to elucidate (Keys *et al.*, 1950).

Attachment and loss

Bowlby, a psychoanalyst working in the context of developmental psychology and object-relations theory, attempts to define and give a meaning to what he sees as the transition and turmoil of adolescence. He takes the view that there are two sets of influences which interact throughout a person's life and whose presence or absence may promote or hinder the development of true self-reliance. The first set of influences, which interact within individuals at all ages and not just during infancy, involves the confidence that standing behind them there are one or more trusted persons who will come to their aid should difficulties arise (Bowlby, 1979, p.103). The second set of influences involves an individual's 'ability to recognize when another person is both trustworthy and willing to provide a base and, second, to collaborate with that person in such a way that a mutually rewarding relationship is initiated and maintained' (p.104).

Bowlby describes how early exploratory behaviour in infants seems to depend on their trust in a secure base, and suggests that not only can infants be classified using observations of their exploratory behaviour, but that premature independence and wariness of others is as little likely to promote later self-reliance as passive dependence. Bowlby's work is helpful because of his insistence that individuals can be both self-reliant and reliant on others. If the terms dependence or independence are used they generally imply value judgements and are rarely specific about whom an individual is dependent upon or independent of. Bowlby's view is that, in speaking of attachment, it is necessary to name the individuals involved, making them available for discussion.

During adolescence, the young person is learning to make use of his or her internal representations of attachment figures and to replace early attachments with new ones. Part of an adolescent's emotional work involves learning to cope with 'the formation, the maintenance, the disruption, and the renewal of attachment relationships' (Bowlby, 1979 p.130). Bowlby describes how 'the threat of loss [of such relationships] gives rise to anxiety and often to anger, and actual loss to the turmoil of feeling that is grief' (p.106).

Anorexia nervosa and adolescents

Classification of the maturational processes of adolescence risks obscuring the ways in which cognitive, affective, behavioural and physiological systems interact. For instance, sexual maturity depends as much on the development of a moral viewpoint as it does on physical development. A moral viewpoint depends on an ability to reflect, think logically and to try out different standpoints. Freedom to think, reflect, discuss and experiment depends in turn on the individual's environment. Pressure on any one component of a system can have a knock-on effect elsewhere in the system that seems quite disproportionate to the original impact.

It is thought that anorexia nervosa provides one way for an adolescent to simplify the processes of development to a few core issues. Food restriction eventually removes many of the destabilizing effects of maturation. The preoccupation with food and the selfishness engendered by starvation have the merit of preventing other disturbing thoughts or awareness of difficulties. A strict morality based on self-discipline and self-judgement removes many problems of moral choice and dilemmas. Both allow maximum conformity to the adolescent's version of parental and family values, while allowing him or her to assert maximum control and apparent independence.

Margo (1985) attempts to identify some factors precipitating the development of anorexia nervosa in adolescence. Using Feighner's criteria (Feighner et al., 1972) he examined forty cases of anorexia nervosa and found an increasing rate of referral which, although the incidence of anorexia nervosa was greater in higher social classes, was associated with an increased proportion of cases in lower social classes. The mean age of onset was 14.3 years, although more than a third of the patients dated onset from before the age of 14. The mean weight loss was 30.5 per cent of premorbid body weight. Nearly a third of the patients complained of being teased about being overweight. The most striking association with onset was the occurrence of major life-events for 60 per cent of patients, ranging from examination failure to parental separation.

Bruch (1981) notes that clinical differentiation of anorexic youngsters is possible on the basis of their sense of personal incompetence and low self-esteem. She ascribes these deficits to early experiences in childhood which distort patients' ability to identify correctly their own feelings and impulses.

Anorexia nervosa and adolescent girls

It is not at all clear how many adolescent girls are at risk of developing anorexia nervosa or other eating disorders. Prediction is made difficult by the multiplicity of identified putative risk factors, and by epidemiological problems of identifying cases in unscreened populations. The instruments used in studying adolescent populations tend to have been developed either for children or adults and may not be valid for adolescents (Mann *et al.*, 1983). The Eating Attitudes Test (Garner and Garfinkel, 1979, 1980; Garner *et al.*, 1982) has been used to screen for clinical and 'subclinical' anorexia nervosa, on the assumption that high EAT scores are associated with both conditions. However, risk factors have been largely identified from the 'patient' rather than general populations (Mann *et al.*, 1983). Additionally, measures of attitudes towards eating conducted across cultures are not necessarily reliable (King and Bhugra, 1989, Snow and Harris, 1989). Johnson-Sabine *et al.* (1988) have shown that it seems likely that, in London schoolgirls at least, abnormal attitudes to eating are contingent on other psychiatric morbidity, and that measures of abnormal eating attitudes are helpful in identifying 'a population at risk for eating disorders', not in diagnosing it (p.620).

The study by Mann *et al.* (1983) identified four diagnostic categories in adolescents: non-dieters, normal dieters, partial syndrome of anorexia nervosa and anorexia nervosa. Johnson-Sabine *et al.* (1988) added bulimia nervosa. Although bulimia is often described as featuring more in late adolescence, and anorexia in early adolescence, Johnson-Sabine *et al.* (1988) suggest that careful epidemiological study may show that bulimia occurs as early in adolescence as anorexia, and that the partial syndrome may be 'an undifferentiated state which can deteriorate into either anorexia or bulimia nervosa' (p.621).

Dietary patterns in teenagers

Huse and Lucas (1984) have confirmed that weight loss in anorexic teenagers is the result of a variety of dietary patterns ranging from bingeing and vomiting to food restriction as implied by Mann *et al.* (1983). The only characteristic shared by dietary patterns was a restriction of caloric intake. Causal relationships between dieting behaviour in teenage schoolgirls and the development of anorexia ner-

vosa have not been reliably demonstrated (Schleimer, 1983). Huon and Brown (1984) found that, in comparing anorexic patients with two groups of youngsters who weighed themselves more or less frequently, the only significant difference was between the least frequent weighers and the patients on the variable of self-esteem.

Diagnosis of anorexia nervosa

Anorexia nervosa is generally diagnosed on the basis of one of two sets of criteria. The DSM–III–R criteria (American Psychiatric Association, 1987) include: 'refusal to maintain body weight over a minimal normal weight for age and height'; 'intense fear of gaining weight or becoming fat'; 'disturbance in the way in which one's body weight, size or shape is experienced'; and amenorrhoea (p.67). Feighner *et al.* (1972) provide five basic criteria: onset before 25 years; body weight loss of 25 per cent or more; food restriction which overrides hunger or coercion to eat; no other physical or psychiatric illness; together with two or more other features from amenorrhoea, lanugo, bradycardia, overactivity, vomiting and bulimia. Russell (1983) describes 'classical' anorexia nervosa as a disorder which 'develops most frequently in adolescent girls after puberty, when it is characterized by a severe and self-induced loss of weight, a cessation of menstruation and a specific psychological disturbance' (p.285). He further defines the psychology as an 'overvalued idea that fatness is a dreadful state. [The patient's] definition of fatness is extremely harsh and she will not let her weight rise above a very low threshold' (p.291).

Aetiology

Piazza *et al.* (1980) supply a conceptual framework for the pathogenesis of anorexia nervosa which includes neuroendocrine vulnerability, disturbed mother–infant relationship, and more severe family disturbance generally. It is not yet possible to be much more specific about the causes of anorexia nervosa, although a great deal of research now exists into these three areas.

Body image

A good deal of evidence appears to support the notion that anorexic patients experience the shape of their body differently from the way the average person does this (Touyz *et al.*, 1984). Clinically it seems that anorexic patients experience their bodies in distorted ways cognitively, emotionally and behaviourally. Body image has been described as a multidimensional construct (Garner *et al.*, 1987). Operating such a construct in order to measure and use it as part of a rationale for treatment, presents a number of problems of bias and distortion of the different dimensions, so that reliability and validity may not be adequate when measures are applied to patients. In any case, as Garner (1981) notes, the direction of causality between anorexia nervosa and body-image, if one exists, is not clear.

Family interaction

Rubin (1986) asserts that deficits in parenting skills and a dysfunctional marital relationship lead to difficulties for children in navigating developmental stages; these difficulties in turn exacerbate parental difficulties. Szmukler *et al.* (1987) demonstrated with a small sample of anorexic patients a high correlation of family interaction with the critical comments component of the expressed emotion rating scale. However, there is some evidence of families of patients with anorexia nervosa who are very close-knit and who assert that they are happier than the average family (Heron and Leheup, 1984).

Representative of some research into anorexic families is a study by Kalucy *et al.* (1977), which looked at 56 families and which, among many other findings, appeared to confirm the commonly held view that anorexia nervosa occurred more often in the higher social classes. They looked closely at the relationship of the parents to each other, but not at that of the siblings to the anorexic family member. They found a high degree of what they termed 'weight pathology' ie., preoccupation with weight, diet and unusual eating patterns in both parents, but especially in the mothers of anorexic adolescents. A significant amount of alcohol abuse was present in fathers but often denied by the family. In a number of families, there was a possibility of separation of the parents which was avoided by their uniting over the illness of their daughter. Kalucy *et al.* (1977) conclude that, although not all families of anorexic adolescents share the features they found in their study and no feature dominated others, a common denominator emerged. 'These families are ill-equipped for and prepare their children inadequately for the adolescent phase of development' (p.394). The reader is referred to Barnes (1984) who provides a scheme of the family life cycle.

Yager (1982) provided a comprehensive review of the literature to date concerning the putative role of family systems in the aetiology of anorexia nervosa. Like Kalucy *et al.* (1977) he regarded a 'typical' anorexic family as being upper middle class, preoccupied with weight, achievement-oriented, and apt to present a window-dressed facade which concealed more or less overt problems of affect, sexuality, impulse control and dependence. However, Yager (1982) noted the methodological deficits of many studies, and accepted that statements about family issues should be conditional on further research. He stressed the need for adequate research into genetic and biological causes of anorexia nervosa.

Other research is beginning to show that family structures and class distribution of people with eating disorders are more complex than originally thought, and that this may be to do with social changes where issues such as anorexia, bulimia, and incest are given a good deal of exposure in mass media, especially television. Martin (1983) has found in a small sample of Canadian families that three subgroups of families containing an anorexic member seem to exist: a group of families who deny any problems; a group who claim to be the 'worst family you have ever seen' (p.59) and a group of families in which the anorexic member appears to 'parade' the disorder.

Family therapy

Minuchin (1974, 1978) is a family systems theorist who pioneered therapy for families containing anorexic adolescents. Minuchin (1978) found that his form of family therapy appears to be associated with a better outcome as long as the anorexic patients are adolescents who come for therapy within a short time of the onset of the anorexia. Goodsitt (1985) found that family therapy is most effective with hospitalized adolescent anorexics who are still living at home. He recommends that it is conducted in the context of stopping visits by the family and restarting contact in the context of therapy.

Russell *et al.* (1987) reported the first controlled trial of family therapy in anorexia nervosa and bulimia nervosa. For adolescents, the most important finding supported Minuchin's assertion that family therapy is more effective where the anorexia was of relatively short duration. However, there were a number of methodological problems with the study which require further investigation, most of which pertain to sample attenuation.

Incest

An increasing number of workers are exploring whether there is a relationship between incest and anorexia nervosa. Sloan and Leichner (1986) give five case illustrations as background to their discussion of whether adolescent sexual conflicts can be explained by actual sexual trauma. They say that the routine investigation of biological and psychosocial factors in patients' anorexia nervosa must include inquiry into such material, so that appropriate therapy for victims of sexual abuse can be incorporated into the treatment regimen.

Genogram

Lewis (1989) suggests that in addition to the standard family genogram designed for displaying the complexities of family relationships and structure, colour coding can be used to demonstrate patterns of roles and characteristics. She gives as an example codings for families with members with eating disorders. Among other characteristics, obsessional personality, substance abuse, incest, disturbance of body image and mental health problems can be colour coded on a genogram by family members. It is desirable that this technique is used by experienced therapists, but the basic genogram

is a useful tool for all disciplines in seeing an identified patient in his or her family context (Hartman and Laird, 1983).

Psychodynamic understanding of anorexia nervosa

The popular idea of psychoanalytic theory (Rycroft, 1968) includes psychoanalysis, ego psychology, individual psychology, analytical psychology, developmental psychology, existential and humanistic therapy. For the purposes of this chapter these are included in the term psychodynamic theory. Selected examples will be illustrated.

Goodsitt (1985), a therapist working with anorexia nervosa from the perspective of self or ego psychology, outlines his concept of self. It includes a structural model which involves emotions and thoughts, needs and desires, forming a hierarchy of values and goals which are both conscious and unconscious. The self's experience of its structure is on a continuum from disorganized or fragmented to organized or cohesive. An individual's sense of self-esteem and worth depends upon where on this continuum he or she experiences her- or himself. Goodsitt (1985) argues that the structure of the self contains a regulating mechanism which balances self-esteem, mood and tension. Perhaps the most important aspect of Goodsitt's explanation is his emphasis on the view that 'anorexia nervosa may occur within a variety of ego or self pathologies' (p.56). However, although there is not a particular anorexic structure of the self, Goodsitt (1985) argues that anorexic people have been unable to develop the self-regulating mechanism which articulates the components of the self, and so do not have any means of identifying and utilizing states of mind and of feeling. Goodsitt shows how anorexic youngsters and their families avoid 'exploring and sharing inner experience' (p.66). Among the anorexic's strategies for doing so is the restriction of food and along with it other forms of nutrition for the inner self. This enables the family to organize its interaction round external representations of inner experience, without having to acknowledge their meaning. The control that anorexics exert over their food intake is a powerfully rewarding substitute for their inner experience of fragmentation. It is therefore virtually impossible for the anorexic to relinquish this sense of mastery by beginning to put on weight, unless the process is initiated and supported by external agencies such as hospital staff.

Bruch's work is probably the best known of the psychodynamic approaches to anorexia nervosa. (Bruch 1978; 1981; 1982). She describes what she calls 'primary anorexia nervosa' to distinguish it from anorexia which is secondary to disorders such as depression or cancer (Bruch, 1982). She asserts that 'although the physical and psychological consequences of the severe malnutrition dominate the manifest clinical picture ... the characteristic psychological disorder is related to underlying deficits in the sense of self, identity, and autonomy' (p.1532).

Feminism and anorexia nervosa

Orbach's (1985) account of anorexia is based on the premise that it predominantly affects girls and women. Her work with anorexic women developed from her therapy of women who were compulsive eaters (Orbach, 1978). Her argument is a complex one which synthesizes psychodynamic and feminist theory.

Orbach postulates the existence of what she calls 'two deeply internalized taboos' which exist in all women. 'One is against the expression of dependency needs, and the other is the taboo against initiating' (p.84). Orbach suggests that apparently dependent behaviour like an inability to manage household repairs masks what she calls 'true dependency needs' which are rarely expressed except in reverse, by having children. A woman attempts to satisfy her own needs through the dependence of the infant upon her. As the girl infant grows up, however, she learns from her mother's example to suppress her own needs. At adolescence, a girl begins to separate from her mother and family and thus to initiate steps towards autonomy, but these steps are thwarted by her experience of ungratified needs which perpetuate her ties to her mother. Orbach cites evidence that girl infants are fed and held for shorter periods than boy infants, learning either restriction or over-feeding during these short intervals. A central

influence on current stereotypes of feminity, families and women's bodies occurred during the post-Second World War period, when women were made redundant from wartime jobs and obliged to return to an idealized version of family life which was disrupted in reality by bereavement and separation. Young women learnt to aim for feelings of success and power by controlling their body size and thus, they hoped the perceptions of them held by those with whom they interact (Orbach, 1985).

Complications of anorexia nervosa in adolescents

A number of studies have investigated the association of anorexia nervosa with other pathology. Dec *et al.* (1987) failed to find evidence of cardiac dysfunction in a small sample of severely emaciated anorexic adolescents. They are careful to point out, however, that electrolyte and metabolic abnormalities do lead to cardiac dysfunction, and that this must be borne in mind when assessing patients who induce vomiting and purging. Reiger *et al.* (1978) found leucopenia in a small sample of anorexic subjects.

Sudden death is a real risk in anorexics with electrolyte disturbance, and the in-patient regimen should be informed by careful attention to safety and by contingency plans for resuscitation should the need arise. Grand mal seizures have occurred in anorexic patients who have insulin-controlled diabetes, and they have been recorded in a hyponatraemic patient who had been drinking large amounts of water to increase her weight (Roberts *et al.*, 1986).

Other metabolic complications include hypercortisolism, thought to originate at hypothalamic level (Raymond, 1987). A topic which is receiving increasing attention is that of the long-term effects of hypo-oestrogenism and its link with osteoporosis. Amenorrhoea which persists from adolescence is associated with severe osteoporosis in comparatively young women and osteoporotic fractures have been recorded in anorexic teenagers (Raymond, 1987). Vertebral bone-loss, and subsequent osteoporosis also been found to be associated with bed-rest in young women with back injuries (Krølner and Toft, 1983). Bed-rest has been commonly used in the first stages of hospitalization of anorexic patients, and so may promote undesirable complications of anorexia nervosa. During a study of voluntary starvation of otherwise healthy men it was found that they excreted calcium at a rate which may be of the order of ten times that calculated on the basis of the body tissue lost (Keys et al., 1950).

Outcome of anorexia nervosa in adolescence

Outcome studies of anorexia nervosa are generally difficult to evaluate because of the lack of standardization of diagnosis especially in relation to severity of the disorder, differences in duration of the follow-up period, small sample sizes and absence of control populations (Steinhausen and Glanville, 1983). In particular, there is a shortage of controlled prospective longitudinal studies of outcome of anorexia nervosa in adolescence. Additionally, the course or natural history of anorexia nervosa if untreated is so variable that outcome of treatment is especially difficult to evaluate (Theander, 1983). Bossert et al. (1988) report that 'the overall treatment outcome of anorexia nervosa, irrespective of the specific treatment method involved, has not improved over recent years' (p.105). A Danish follow-up of 151 anorexic adolescents between four and twenty-two years after treatment showed that about half were free of symptoms while about a quarter were still anorexic despite treatment. In view of the large number of patients with chronic anorexia nervosa this study raises particular questions about the natural history of the disorder (Tolstrup et al., 1985). Steinhausen and Glanville (1983) found impairment and continuing symptoms in up to two thirds of female patients followed up about ten years after anorexia nervosa in adolescence. It was clear that for a large proportion of the sample studied that the long-term prognosis was poor. Other studies indicate that recovery from anorexia nervosa cannot be correlated with any specific treatments (Steinhausen and Glanville, 1983; Bassøe and Esklund, 1982). Morgan et al. (1983) confirm that poor prognostic features for adolescents include the duration of illness before referral, previous personality problems and family

conflict. They suggest that long-term follow-up is necessary to monitor the chronic nature of the disorder. Crisp (1984) asserts that a better prognosis results from interventions aimed at treating the long-term causes of anorexia nervosa. Bassøe and Esklund (1982) indicate that a better outcome exists in patients who seek treatment soon after onset of their anorexia nervosa.

Criteria for admission to hospital

Carino and Chmelko (1983) cite as their criteria for admission 25 per cent or more loss of body weight; electrolyte imbalance; excessive tension within the family; suicide risk; obsessive-compulsive symptoms; and lack of cooperation with outpatient treatment.

Inpatient treatment of anorexia nervosa in adolescents

In the nineteenth century both Marcé and Gull (Silverman, 1989; Gull, 1894) recommended that the anorexic girl should be removed from the influence of her family, who were thought likely to undermine the authority of the physician, even when they felt they were working toward the same goal of ensuring that the anorexic ate and put on weight. Vandereycken (1985) calls this approach which is still favoured in some treatment centres 'parentectomy' (p.415).

Although the model of the physician's (or the multidisciplinary clinical team's) authority can be strongly challenged, it does have many social supports. Orbach (1985) has found that anorexic women need three to five years of individual psychotherapy to initiate and maintain changes away from their anorexic behaviour. The structure of medical and hospital services in the UK is not geared to providing such care and private psychotherapy is expensive. Further, the fundamental theoretical and political differences between Orbach's model and the conventional psychiatric model seem to represent a wider crisis in psychiatry as a whole (Williams, 1986). Attempts to adopt a version of Orbach's model in a conventional psychiatric setting risk amplifying the existing potential for staff conflict involved in caring for anorexic patients. There is evidence that a coherent treatment programme with a long follow-up does benefit a substantial number of anorexic patients (Morgan and Russell, 1975).

Russell (1977) suggested that 'the most immediately effective method of treatment is simply to admit the patient to hospital assuming that a basic level of care and understanding of the illness are available'. He puts nurses at the centre of a general programme of management which he emphasizes does not constitute a 'specific method of treatment for anorexia nervosa' (p.280).

Vandereycken (1985) gives an account of changing treatment philosophies over a number of years in his unit. He usefully illustrates how interaction with anorexic patients themselves, between the staff and with other patients, leads to changes in a treatment regimen. In addition, he carefully monitored all patients on a long-term basis, so that what he calls a multifaceted group approach evolved. He emphasizes that anorexic patients are deliberately treated in a mixed unit, and that adolescent patients are treated with older patients in order to avoid encouraging an 'anorexic identity' of which some patients are proud. Older patients can also benefit from the presence of adolescents, who allow them to explore aspects of their own development which have been troubled.

Rollins and Blackwell (1968) provide an account of inpatient treatment of adolescents with anorexia nervosa, based partly on Winnicott's (1965) theory of 'maturational processes and the facilitating environment'. As indicated elsewhere in this chapter, Rollins has expanded her conceptual framework for anorexia nervosa, but Winnicott's theories of holding and Bion's (1970) related theories of containing remain an essential underpinning of any attempt to provide a psychodynamically informed milieu for anorexic youngsters.

Rollins and Blackwell (1968) assert that the ward or unit must provide a corrective emotional experience for youngsters who have not navigated developmental stages satisfactorily, and who tend to be consumed with anger that they have difficulty in expressing in words. One aim of the milieu is 'to provide an atmosphere in which the manipulation, controlling anger and rage of the anorectic youngster can be expressed, but with a therapist who can stand firm against the onslaught' (p.85). The therapist who can stand firm may be a psychotherapist or may be a primary nurse or other key worker (Piazza *et al.*, 1980).

Harding (1985) asserts that short-term 'treatment goals for anorexia nervosa are to restore optimal nutritional status and prevent recurrence of the disorder' (p.276) by means of nutritional therapy, psychotherapy and family therapy, either on an out-patient or in-patient basis. Long-term goals include maintenance of optimal nutritional status, physically and psychological maturation and resolution of underlying conflicts. Hospitalization is indicated in the presence of severe emaciation and electrolyte imbalance. She includes among treatment methods weight gain and stabilization followed by psychotherapy; correcting a distorted body image; behaviour modification; teamwork; one-to-one nursing supervision and primary nursing.

Chambers and Yong (1985) provide a British perspective on in-patient management shared by a psychiatric and a general nursing unit in a children's hospital. They emphasize the importance of joint multidisciplinary meetings, attended by key representatives, to maintain consistency and to avoid confusion.

Williams (1982) describes in considerable detail a milieu therapy programme in western Australia. She recommends that the nursing team consists of qualified nurses specializing in eating disorders, and that it is autonomous and relatively small. The two aspects of the treatment programme are aimed at restoring physical health and correcting psychological distortions. Her recommendations are now in some doubt because of their emphasis on prolonged bed rest, but her account of the milieu and of specific nursing interventions are useful.

Bryant and Kopeski (1986) use Gordon's (1982) functional health patterns to outline the principles of nursing care for patients with eating disorders. They recommend that food intake is negotiated with the dietician, but should approximate to 'three, balanced high-fibre meals, adequate hydration, and monitored exercise' (p.60). They assert that 'reaching target weight is the most difficult goal for the eating disorder client to accept and work towards' (p.62). They emphasize safety not only in terms of suicide prevention, which is advocated by most authors, but also in terms of anticipating violent expression of 'intense feelings of anger, abandonment, and fear of rejection' (p.64).

The multidisciplinary clinical team

Rubin (1986) recommends that the multidisciplinary clinical team agrees between itself the limits to be imposed on the anorexic patient and that these limits are plainly communicated to the patient; that all team members observe the agreed limits; that the patient knows what the consequences of breaking limits are, and that there is a schedule of reinforcement.

Carino and Chmelko (1983) recommend a holistic, multidisciplinary approach, based on a conception of the patient as a 'biopsychosocial being who is in continuous interaction with his or her environment' (p.349). They provide a very complex set of nursing interventions summarized in a useful checklist, which includes nursing supervision of meals for 60–90 minutes after eating and daily weighing after the bladder is voided. Carino and Chmelko identify eleven problem areas in addition to the main nursing programme. The way in which anorexia nervosa overwhelms the life of the anorexic person is vividly illustrated in this paper, along with the difficulties in selecting and agreeing priorities.

In their account of a multidimensional psychotherapeutic treatment programme for anorexic adolescents, Boyle et al. (1981) provide synopses of the roles of the different members of the multidisciplinary clinical team caring for anorexic youngsters, describing the role of the primary nurse as pivotal to the core of the nursing as well as of the multidisciplinary team. They describe a programme of withdrawal and restoration and privileges based on target weight gain and contained within a treatment agreement between patient and staff. The responsibilities of the primary nurse include monitoring and recording intake and output, daily weight and vital signs, and liaising between the patient, family and other staff concerning the effectiveness of the current treatment plan. Although after refeeding many of the issues to be addressed are psychological, they recommend that behavioural objectives are maintained in the context of a programme of individual psychotherapy, group therapy, family therapy, occupational therapy and group therapy for parents. They stress, in common with other writers, that weight gain alone is rarely enough to ensure recovery from anorexia nervosa. Unfortunately, there is little evidence to support estimations of the duration of time necessary to consolidate interventions other than those directed at weight gain before the patient leaves hospital.

Horne and Gallen (1987) describe the difficulties which result from the multiplicity of interventions required in the treatment of patients with anorexia nervosa. It is not necessarily clear in a multidisciplinary setting which staff are responsible for which interventions. This can have adverse effects on the formation of an effective therapeutic alliance with the patient. Horne and Gallen (1987) recommend that the role of each member of the multidisciplinary team is clearly defined and kept within specified boundaries. The patient's attempts to categorize staff into roles which fit with his or her experiences of other people are thus balanced by a secure and confident division of roles by staff who are less likely to be drawn into re-enactments of parental and other family conflicts.

Role of the nurse

Because anorexic patients tend to be admitted when their weight and endocrine function are severely compromised by continuing dietary restriction, the severity of these physical complications risk imposing on all disciplines a so-called medical model approach. Nurses especially are apt to see this approach as involving physical interventions which are exclusive of and take priority over psychological interventions. As a result they tend to feel unable to contribute a distinctive theoretical slant to a team management plan which is dominated by the medical urgency of the anorexic's condition. In anorexia nervosa the patient has effectively separated mind from body, becoming unable to express or represent thoughts and feelings in words. In the patient's view, the food offered by the staff is physical nutrition only, and not food for thought. This view may be shared by the nurses looking after the patient.

Schlemmer and Barnett (1977) describe aspects of the nurses' role in a comparison of treatments for anorexia nervosa in the USA. Unfortunately no evaluative data are presented. However, these aspects include room searches; a dietician-controlled diet; a refusal to discuss any aspect of food; prevention of food hoarding; prevention of food disposal; limiting time in the bathroom; limiting time associating with other patients; limiting visitors; ensuring that patients void before being weighed; frequent staff meetings for the purpose of ventilating feelings of anger and frustration; consistent following by all staff of treatment programmes and reviewing non-judgementally with patients their behaviour. They hypothesize that anorexic patients behave in a more tricky way the more restrictions are placed on them. McNamara (1982) also recommends primary nursing along with good inter-shift communication; adequate staffing levels; multidisciplinary management meetings; dietician monitored refeeding; joining the patient in eating a meal; titrating weight gain against calorie intake; daily weighing; restriction of activity and monitoring of suicide risk. McNamara (1982) asserts that although 'there are no hard and fast rules' for nursing the anorexic patient, it is possible to identify potential problems which recur. Perhaps because of the widespread social acceptance of preoccupation with weight and diet, anorexic patients are able to challenge nurses' sense of their own level of mental health, and can intimidate them into uncertainty and inconsistency in care and management. Misik (1981) suggests some answers to challenging questions by anorexic patients.

Lilly and Sanders (1987) provide four case reports which illustrate the false starts that nursing programmes may have to tolerate before a regimen suited to the needs of an individual patient can be decided. Their anorexic patients are treated in general psychiatric units and a 'generic eating disorder protocol' is provided which is changed according to patients' needs.

Clark (1983) suggests that female nurses are subject to the same social pressures as anorexic women. These pressures are said by Schwartz *et al.* (1982) to amount to a 'new cultural obsession: the relentless pursuit of thinness' (p.20).

Wooley and Wooley (1982) went so far as to say that the Beverly Hills Diet was the mass marketing of anorexia nervosa. Palmer (1980) notes that the nurse who has experience of dieting to lose weight 'may be torn between empathy for the anorexic's fear of becoming fat, and annoyance at her childish behaviour' (p.102). Clark (1983) quotes a selection of nurses' comments made to anorexic patients, including 'I'm on a diet too, but it doesn't work that well for me!' (p.6). Schwartz *et al.* (1982) note that the range of attitudes, values and beliefs shared by normal-weight women with anorexic women is as yet unmeasured. Clark (1983) warns that the resulting mixed feelings experienced by nurses looking after anorexic patients potentially undermine their ability to maintain a therapeutic relationship which is, by definition, professional. When, therefore, Crisp (1980) advocates that trained nurses who are 'still in touch with their own adolescent struggles' offer 'friendship' to anorexic patients, with whom they can share experience, he is suggesting a course of action that may not be to the advantage either of the patient or the nurse. Other writers make similar recommendations (McNamara 1982). Clark (1983) makes the extremely important point that, quite independently of any supposed empathic process, identification with patients expressed in comments such as 'when you get out of here you won't have a thing to wear', acts to reinforce patients' anorexic behaviour.

The role of uncontrolled reinforcement in ward settings received a good deal of attention during early developments of behaviour therapy, when investigators were interested in seeing how nurses' behaviour contributed to the maintenance of undesirable behaviour by patients. Following Skinner's (1957) definition of verbal behaviour Ayllon and Haughton (1964) suggested that social reaction to particular kinds of verbal behaviour could act as a reinforcer which would maintain that behaviour. They found that patients' undesirable behaviour often received a good deal of attention from nurses, whether in sympathetic listening, attempts to argue them out of mistaken or delusional beliefs, or expressions of impatience. They trained psychiatric nurses to observe and identify types of undesirable verbal behaviour, and then to withhold social attention (positive reinforcement) to that behaviour. The nurses were asked to record observations over 15–20 days, before selecting behaviour in which they could intervene by withholding positive reinforcement. Withholding social attention consisted of looking away, acting as if interested in something else, appearing busy with something, appearing distracted, looking bored, appearing to attend to something else in the ward. Ayllon and Haughton's conclusion is a strong plea for hospital staff to recognize the influence the environment has upon patients' behaviour, and the ways in which inconsistent approaches by different staff members can have the effect of strengthening and increasing undesired behaviours even when all staff are apparently agreed on the goals of treatment.

Staff relationships

Clark (1983) insists that the nurse who feels that she identifies with an anorexic patient to the extent of questioning the treatment programme has an obligation to share her doubts with the rest of the team and not with the patient. Nurses, particularly in the early stages of their experience, can often find themselves agreeing to share and keep secrets with patients, basing this on a mistaken view of the ethic of confidentiality.

Sansone *et al.* (1988) conducted a study designed to see whether nurses working in an in-patient unit ran any particular risks as a result of the setting. They assumed two areas of potential difficulty: firstly, the need to have a good psychodynamic understanding of such patients; and secondly, the ability to deploy a range of 'sophisticated interpersonal skills' in order to maintain a 'consistent balance of emotional support coupled with nonjudgemental limit setting' (p.126). They measured mood, weight, eating attitudes, job satisfaction and attitudes to patients comparing the nurses working with patients with eating disorders with nurses working in other areas. Because of the small sample and other methodological difficulties the results must be interpreted with caution, but the authors

claim that nurses are not at any particular risk on their measures, and attribute this to the team-building processes in the eating disorders unit.

This fragmentation of thought, feeling and action ensures that a ward where anorexics are treated is a fertile setting for what have been termed multiple transference phenomena. Horne and Gallen (1987) advocate a strict division of roles along traditionally defined lines, leaving psychotherapeutic interventions to a psychotherapist. However, this view begs the question of the definition of psychotherapy. A more productive framework divides psychotherapy into four categories or level, allowing the multidisciplinary clinical team to allocate roles and responsibilities among its members without confusing what the nurses are doing with what is being done by the other disciplines (Cawley, 1976; Ritter, 1988; Ritter, 1989).

Weight

In order to estimate the severity of weight loss the premorbid weight must be known. The procedure of expressing the degree of starvation in an individual by reference to average body weights 'may be grossly misleading' (Keys *et al.*, 1950, p.86). It is not clear how much weight is lost with what caloric insufficiency. There is some evidence that weight loss is greatest in those who are fattest at the beginning of reduction of caloric intake. There is also evidence that in anorexia nervosa a much greater degree of weight loss is tolerated than in other forms of starvation, and Orbach states that she does not regard a stably low weight as a medical emergency (Keys *et al.*, 1950; Orbach, 1985).

The target body weight of anorexic youngsters is often based upon the weight at which menstruation is thought likely to start. Frisch and McArthur (1974) provides scales for calculating this weight. It is possible to ask the patient how much she weighed when she last had periods, but this information is not necessarily reliable. As Frisch and McArthur point out, amenorrhoea occurs for a number of reasons in addition to weight loss, and must be properly investigated.

The position reported by Russell and Mezey

(1962) has not greatly changed. Our information about weight restoration and dietary content for anorexia patients is flawed and incomplete. Correction of undernourishment in subjects who have starved involuntarily or in a research programme is not necessarily comparable with the same process in anorexia. One difficulty in researching high-calorie diets is that anorexic patients are apt not to co-operate with such diets, and with the repeated measures of their nutritional status. General guidance about calorie intake can be offered, but in general, it seems that treatment centres develop their own approach, based on an overall treatment philosophy as much as on specific research about refeeding.

Goodsitt (1985) recommends a target weight of 90 per cent of 'ideal body weight' at a rate of 1 lb a week. Orr (1979) recommends $2\frac{1}{2}$ to 3 lb per week. Misik (1981)))) recommends $\frac{1}{2}$ lb per day. Boyle, Koff and Gudas (1981) suggest an unspecified daily target weight. However, as Wright (1986) indicates in an empathetic though seriously limited review of some of the perceptual changes in anorexia nervosa, many problems of compliance and motivation underlie a process seen by some nurses, as well as by some anorexics, as akin to fattening livestock. Williams (1982) puts into perspective one aspect of weight gain which distresses some patients and nurses. The 'patients tend to look plump, but they quickly lose this plump appearance as muscle develops and there is a general distribution of the weight to allow full activities' (p.40).

Russell (1977) uses life assurance tabulations of average body weight as a guide for target weights (Diem and Lentner, 1970). When weight gain starts it is likely to be rapid. Russell (1977) shows the weight charts of two adolescent girls aged 15 which indicate a gain of 12.6 kg in 31 days in one case and 15.5 kg in the other.

The rest of the chapter will use a case study of a 15-year-old patient called Kate, in order to illustrate, in practical terms, some of the theoretical material discussed so far. The admission sheet (Figure 11.2) is designed to introduce Kate and to provide a context for her treatment in hospital. The genogram (Figure 11.3) is designed to place Kate in the context of her family and to draw the reader's attention to the interaction between the person with anorexia nervosa and apparently unrelated events in her family.

Chronology of Kate's admission

3 January – 2 February

Kate continued to lose weight and there were several confrontations with the nurses.

At first, the team decided to assess Kate's needs and problems before embarking on a definitive treatment plan. In the psychiatrist's opinion the nursing assessment would decide how the team's plan would be conducted. An initial assessment period of three weeks was planned, during which the nurses planned to try to get to know Kate, to make a working relationship with her, to try to obtain Kate's view of her current predicament along with her family's view, and to make as full a physical assessment as possible (complementing the doctors' investigations of her physical state) to rule out any underlying physical disease causing weight loss, and to assess her family situation and her current mental state.

Evaluation

Problem 1

Kate has tended to try to talk to her nurses at times when they are not able to stay with her, for example, at meal times, at times when groups are scheduled, and when nurses are meant to be in staff meetings. She complains that the nurses fob her off all the time and that they are not really interested in her. At other times she goes to her room and lies on her bed listening to her personal stereo. As a result the nurses feel that either they must reinforce behaviour to which they object (Kate detaining them from other work) or they must withhold positive reinforcement for behaviour which is, after all, stated as desirable in the care plan.

PATIENT'S NAME   Kate Brown   HOSPITAL NUMBER   246810

Next of kin [address and telephone]
Mother: Mrs Brown, 4 Rose Cottages, Mill Lane, Beckenham
Tel: 671 0060

Person to be contacted in emergency [address and telephone]
Mother [as above]

Primary and associate nurses
Diane Michael, Rory O'Neill, Rosie Carter

Reason for admission
Referred by local psychiatrist after six months out-patient treatment. Kate has lost about 40 per cent of her previous weight. She is refusing to eat. She has been admitted for investigations to establish the causes of her weight loss, and to start a re-feeding programme if necessary.

Patient's view of current needs/problems
'I don't know what all the fuss is about'
'Why don't you all leave me alone?'
'I have to study for my GCSE's'

Relatives'/friends'/ view of current needs/problems
Kate's mother says she can't cope with trying to comply with Kate's vegetarian diet and strict rules which effectively means she has stopped eating. She has been told by a colleague at work that Kate could die. She blames her recent divorce for Kate's illness.

Safety towards self/others
Mother thinks Kate is suicidal. She has been yelling a lot lately at the family and slapped her younger sister 2 days ago.

Nursing summary
Kate is nearly 16. She is still at school, and has been losing weight since she started dieting two years ago. She has been a vegetarian for four years. Although father left home about four years ago there is some question whether he abused Kate sexually before that. She is quite hostile to the nurses. Kate may be bingeing and vomiting, and is to be on an accompanied pass and observed closely. Safety care plan implemented.

Consultant	Bed state	Keys	TPR/BP	Urinalysis	Certificate
Dr Smith	Yes. Main dormitory	Yes	95.6/38 90/50	Tr. Ketones Tr. Protein	See Welfare Officer

Hospital no registered	Property	Ward	Weight	Missing person form	Religion
Yes	Checked	A	25.4 kg	Yes	Christian

Admitting nurse [name in capitals and signature]				Date	
Diane Michael				3/1/19–	

Figure 11.2   Admission sheet

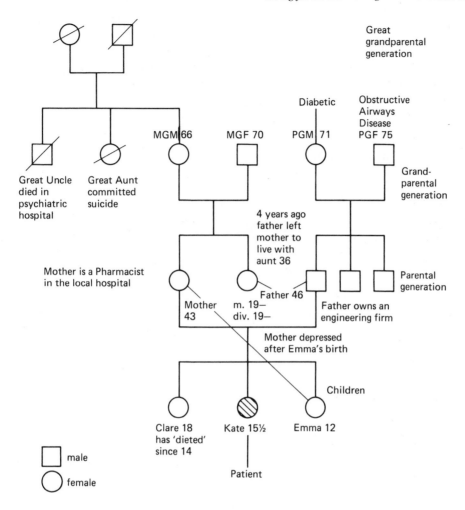

Figure 11.3 Kate's family genogram

Problems	Patient Action	Nursing Intervention
1. Kate finds it difficult to talk to people and say what she needs.	Kate will initiate one conversation per shift with her primary or associate nurses, depending who is on duty.	Kate's nurses will provide positive verbal reinforcement when Kate initiates conversation.
2. Kate does not know what she wants from her admission to hospital	Kate will think about what she wants and what she would like to achieve	Kate's primary and associate nurses will discuss and negotiate with Kate her goals for this admission.

Figure 11.4 First care plan short-term goals

Problem 2

Kate spends a good deal of time writing in her diary, but is unwilling to share this with her nurses. She continues to say that she does not know what she wants.

Nursing assessment at the end of Kate's first week in hospital

Self care

Kate showers twice a day. Her clothes are big on her, and she always seems cold. She carries a cushion everywhere with her.

Sleep

Kate sleeps very irregularly. She says she wakes at about 5 am every morning. She also has difficulty going to sleep at night. She says, 'I cannot stop thinking'. She is prescribed 10 mg of temazepam every night, but the night staff think she is concealing them. She gets up at 6 am and stands and looks out of the window for an hour or longer if uninterrupted. (She says she is looking at the clouds.)

Appetite

Kate always needs prompting to go to the canteen. When she showers, she takes so long that she misses breakfast if unnoticed by the nurses. If chased to breakfast she may take so long about it that she misses the morning group. She sits and stares at a plate of cornflakes going soggy, two slices of bread, a spoonful of marmalade, and a cup of tea. She often disappears at midday, missing lunch if possible. She sits and stares at her food. She sometimes disappears before supper. Sometimes she brings her food back to the ward, saying it is too crowded in the canteen. When she attempts to wash up her crockery and cutlery after meals, she spends twenty or thirty minutes washing a plate and knife and fork. She dithers about whether to eat or throw away things like an apple core. Sometimes the ward cleaner or nursing assistants get impatient with her and argue with her about her slowness. This often means that she eats even less.

Occupying her time

Kate does not speak much to the other patients. She spends her time reading, listening to her personal stereo, playing cards (Patience), and writing in her diary. She prefers to stay lying on her bed, though she will sit in the main ward if asked to. She enjoys going out for walks.

Mood

According to Kate's self-evaluation, she says, 'I have not been able to cry, but feel as if I am suppressing everything. I have been refusing to let myself cry as this is a great weakness and a way of losing control of myself. On some occasions I have tried to sit down and write how I am feeling but have not been successful as I cannot concentrate when I am in that state'. She says she often feels panicky. When this happens, she feels she must 'clam up' or lose control.

Weight

Kate has refused to be weighed.

Social competence

Kate does not mix a great deal with other patients. She seems to find it easier to talk to nurses, as long as they make the first approach. She says she misses school where 'everyone knew me'. She looks after two old ladies in the ward. Sometimes she socializes with other patients briefly in the evenings and she can play backgammon, but she usually spends a long time pottering round her bed sorting out her belongings looking at books, writing. Often she does not get to bed before midnight or later, and sits on the edge of her bed or on her own in the day room.

Groups

Kate avoids the ward groups if she can, and as yet has not spoken. If she comes she always sits in the same chair and curls up with her special cushion. Sometimes she takes so long to get dressed and to have breakfast that she comes to the group without washing and in her night attire. If one of the nurses asks her to get dressed before coming to the group, Kate leaves and does not return. She goes and lies on her bed.

Family and visitors

Kate's mother visits nearly every other day, bringing clean clothes and bottles of fruit juice. She and Kate sit in silence a lot of the time, and her mother becomes quite tearful. Kate's father visited at the weekend with her aunt. Kate's father is a handsome man who strikingly resembles Kate. Kate's aunt was very well turned-out with highlighted and permed hair and plenty of make-up – 'power-dressing'. Her preliminary words to Kate, with no greeting were, 'What's this new trick, hunched up like that? What are you doing that for?' Kate was standing with her hands in pockets, shoulders hunched up to ears. Kate's father was mostly silent and sat with his arm round Kate while her aunt conducted a virtual monologue with her. After they left Kate went to the radio and danced on her own for twenty minutes or so to the records being played.

Summary

Kate appears to have settled reasonably well into the ward and says she likes the system of nursing. She does not mix because she says she 'is of no value and not worthy of attention'. I feel that she is implementing her care plan by tending to approach nurses other than her primary and associate nurses, and think this needs monitoring closely. She has received a letter from a teacher at school. Her relationship with her mother is very strained, and her relationship with her father seems quite disturbed. The main problem is that she is eating very little and seems quite adept at avoiding food. As she has refused to be weighed, I cannot say definitely if she has lost more weight, but think that this is so. I don't think she abuses laxatives or vomits because she is able to avoid food completely if given the opportunity. She is low in mood, and her Wakefield score indicates that she is depressed.

An account by Rory, her associate nurse, of an incident ten days after admission

Kate refused to go down for breakfast this morning. She bolted for the ward door shouting that she must get out and we were not to stop her. Anna and Mike (staff nurse and nursing assistant) shut the door and explained to Kate that we were all concerned about her safety and would implement the Nurse's Holding Power. She became very angry and ran to the bathroom, locking herself in and refusing to talk to any of her nurses. The duty doctor was called to assess her, and she eventually came out of the bathroom and met with the doctor for an hour. She agreed not to leave the ward unaccompanied and went to her room. At lunchtime she again refused to go to the canteen. I was not prepared to leave her in the ward because I felt that I would be unable to supervise her safely. She eventually agreed to go to the canteen and ate a small amount of lunch. Di met with Kate after lunch and praised her for going with me to the canteen. I offered to take her for a walk this afternoon, and we went out for half an hour. Kate told me that she finds that if she can control her eating she does not get angry and so cannot hurt anybody. I pointed out to her that she had become very angry with me at lunch time. She agreed and said that the only reason she had not hit me was that she was afraid I would hit her back. She then apologized for becoming angry with me. Even though I explained that it was okay for her to feel angry at me she would not accept this and said she had to direct it inwards towards herself.

Signed: Rory O'Neill

The ward round held three weeks after Kate's admission was a tense occasion. Kate was insisting on going on weekend leave in order to be with her mother on her mother's birthday. She packed her weekend bag ostentatiously during OT time on Friday morning before the ward round. She was planning to cook supper for her mother that evening and to go out shopping on Saturday. Kate was furious during the ward round when told by the consultant that he would not agree to weekend leave. She stormed out and locked herself in the bathroom.

After a long discussion it was decided to have a cooling-off period over the weekend and to implement treatment for Kate's anorexia the following Monday. Kate's primary nurse, the charge nurse, the senior registrar and the registrar were asked to agree the treatment plan with Kate, and to inform her mother.

2 February – 16 February

The team decided to start a programme designed to treat Kate's anorexia. She was transferred to a side room. After her initial assessment, weekly haematological and blood chemistry measures were discontinued, as the staff were confident that she was not vomiting or using laxatives. Kate was asked to stay in her room. She attended the ward groups, held twice daily; a religious seminar held by the chaplains once a week; hospital chapel on Sundays; and a modified occupational therapy programme of relaxation and music appreciation. The other patients visited her room at the ward's usual visiting times, after discussion with Kate and the nurses in the ward groups. Kate was asked to negotiate visits by a maximum of two people a day, and to restrict her use of the ward telephone to one call a day.

Evaluation

Kate has achieved her objective. However, she is not carrying out all her agreed actions. She is talking throughout her meals, so that she is eating for up to an hour and a half at a time. The nurses do not feel able to disattend to her talking and have been arguing with her about her food. There is also some conflict between the nurses and between the nurses and the registrar about Kate's programme, as Kate has been complaining to him about the food. Kate has refused to be weighed.

The care plan is to continue for another seven days.

16 February – 17 March

Kate gained weight rapidly (Figure 11.6). As a result of the nurses' problems with Kate's persistence in talking about food, they role-played the various ways of disattending it. Some felt more comfortable reading, some knitted, others practised looking distracted. The important element was that they put away these distractions in order to listen to Kate when she talked about matters other than

food. Gradually Kate started to eat her meals more quickly and to talk to her nurses about things ranging from the books she was reading, through to religion, and to what had led up to her admission to hospital.

This work by the nurses (tailoring the form and content of their relationship with Kate to her needs) is Level P2 psychotherapy (Cawley, 1976; Ritter, 1968; Ritter, 1989). In Kate's case their work was informed by the psychodynamic understanding of anorexia nervosa that was held in the ward.

In a ward where psychoanalytic theory is used to inform nursing practice, and where patients are treated by psychotherapists, it is essential that there is a model which allows the different disciplines to discriminate between their roles and responsibilities for aspects of the patient's care. Cawley's 'levels of psychotherapy' provide a theoretical framework whereby nurses develop and use therapeutic relationships with patients which complement the interventions of other staff. The four components of this framework are levels P1 to P4 psychotherapy. In level P2 psychotherapy, the nurse–patient relationship is the vehicle for the delivery of care which is not only tailored to the needs of the patient but also takes into account the effects of the relationship upon the nurses themselves. Because 'the objectives are as diverse as the patients' problems' (Ritter, 1988, p.111), nurses working at level P2 psychotherapy need a structured framework which gives them the confidence to manage patients who provoke much anxiety.

The nature of anorexia nervosa means that nursing care which is designed to help the patient put on weight, actually triggers enormous stress and often hostility in the anorexic patient. Nurses can interpret this distress as a product of their interaction with the patient and as an onslaught on their personal effectiveness. The risk is that the communication by the patient of her dread of relinquishing control over her weight is misunderstood as non-compliance.

Because of her obvious distress, the nurses felt it was important to communicate to her that they understood her preoccupation with food to be both a product of her starving herself, and also a sign of her wish to retain her control over her frightening

Need	Objective	Patient action	Nursing intervention
Kate needs to regain a body weight that is acceptable for her age and height.	Supervised by a nurse at mealtimes, Kate will eat three meals and three snacks a day for the next seven days.	Kate will remain in her room unless she has scheduled activities in the ward, or in the chapel.	Kate's nurses will bring her snacks at coffee times, tea-time and bed-time.
		She will choose her meals from the hospital menu provided.	Kate's nurse will provide her with the hospital menu so that she can choose her meals.
		She will eat her meals in the company of a nurse.	They will sit with Kate while she eats her meals and snacks and remain with her for an hour after she has finished eating.
		She will refrain from talking to the nurse while she is eating.	Kate's nurse will ignore Kate talking during her meals unless it is about topics other than food or weight.
		She will agree to be weighed once a week by her primary nurse.	Kate's primary nurse will weigh her once a week on the same day at the same time.

Figure 11.5 Second care plan.

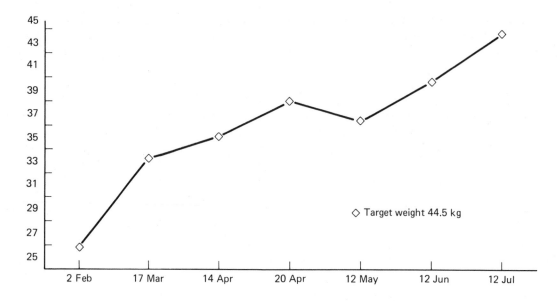

Figure 11.6   Kate's weight chart.

problems. The nurses were asked to explain to Kate that they understood how severe her anxiety must have been when she first decided to restrict her food intake. The enterprise of weight gain was to be a joint venture in which the nurses took over control of her food, and in doing so would remove her sense of control. This would inevitably mean that underlying problems would surface, and she would feel very distressed not to be able to apply her own methods of controlling them. The work of the nurses was to help Kate to find new ways of dealing with her needs to depend on others, to face her problems of rivalry and sexuality, and to allow her family to find its own way of dealing with its problems (Jackson, 1981).

Kate told the nurses that her problems started when she was aged 13. She attends a co-educational school. At that time she felt her breasts developed too quickly for her age, and that the boys made fun of her. She weighed 46 kg, with a height of 150 cm. She felt that her build was abnormal, that the lower half of her body was out of proportion to the upper half, and that her legs were too long and her shoulders were too broad, emphasizing her large breasts. Her periods started when she

was 12. They were irregular and she always felt embarrassed by them, feeling that the boys could tell when she was menstruating. Her periods stopped altogether when she was 14. She did not tell anyone that this was the case, and would often complain of dysmenorrhoea at school, using this and other reasons to avoid organized sports. Paradoxically she became interested in jogging and embarked on a running programme which (unknown to her mother and teachers) led her to run up to ten miles a day starting at 6 am.

Kate also told the nurses that when she was eleven, shortly after her father went to live with her aunt, he took the children on holiday in a self-catering villa in Marbella. This had been unpleasant and embarrassing. Kate and Claire had felt guilty about their mother and angry with Emma for enjoying herself. Kate returned to her mother's home and became more preoccupied with eating healthily. Neither she nor her mother made any connection between this and the holiday.

17 March – 14 April
Kate's weight gain started to slow down (Figure 11.6). She was eating less and appeared to be becoming more obsessional. The nurses were con-

cerned, but felt they were losing touch with her, and felt unable to find out what was wrong. For the time being the care plan continued.

14 April – 7 May

Kate suddenly gained 2 kg in twenty-four hours, and appeared quite bloated (Figure 11.6). It was found that she was drinking large quantities of water. She would comply with nurses requests to come out of the bathroom or kitchen, but would sneak back. When they were locked, she was found drinking from the cleaner's mop bucket. She had been neglecting herself and picking at spots and scabs on her body. After interviews with the ward doctors and a team discussion she was thought to be psychotic, and she was given oral trifluoperazine 2 mg in the morning and 2 mg at night. When there was some doubt whether she was swallowing tablets, she was given her medication in liquid form. She returned to normal drinking and her mental state improved after about three weeks.

In retrospect, it seemed that part of the precipitant for her psychosis was the departure of the registrar, whom Kate had been seeing once a week, and to whom she had become very attached and with whom she had been able to discuss the 'emergence of her sexual feelings and the guilt it had always caused her' (Jackson, 1981). At the same time, several patients were discharged and the senior registrar left. Kate's self-reproaches and her self-humiliation seemed to be linked with her guilt about the breakup of the family, and to earlier more primitive experiences in infancy. The loss of the attachment figures in the ward did not at that time allow her to become aware of and deal with the losses in her life other than by becoming psychotically overwhelmed.

The nurses maintained their emphasis on re-feeding Kate, keeping her safe and helping her look after herself. She herself felt unable to handle any emotional contact with other people. Although her nurses refrained from digging in when they talked with her, they found they had to be quite confrontational about maintaining Kate's programme of meals and snacks and her other activities.

7 May – 8 June

As Kate's psychosis resolved the team decided to ask a family therapist to meet with Kate's family.

The first meeting was with Kate's family of origin, but her father refused to attend after two meetings. Kate, her mother and sisters attended all subsequent sessions. During the same period Kate's rehabilitation programme started, headed by the occupational therapist.

Kate had become vegetarian after the holiday with her father and aunt apparently because of a television programme about conditions of animals being slaughtered. She had told her mother that she could obtain sufficient calories from beans and rice, and started to avoid eggs, cheese and milk. She started cooking her own meals. She also justified this by saying that as her mother worked it was not fair to expect her to cook when she came in. If her mother cooked for her she would calculate the protein and carbohydrate content of the food and leave what she felt was surplus to her needs. Kate's mother felt unable to challenge her. Kate would stay in her room apparently watching her own television or doing homework. Gradually she became agitated about her schoolwork, spending long periods of time in her room with her school books, and would scream at her mother if she asked about homework. Kate would pack her own lunches to eat at school. She would isolate herself at meal times.

In the family sessions Kate revealed how in the early stages of her food restriction she would feel so hungry after eating her diet lunch that she would go to the local shop and buy chocolate bars and crisps and eat them as quickly as possible. The subsequent nausea and disgust with herself made her withdraw further from friends and family and she would restrict the amount in her lunch pack even further. Her best friend from junior school became attached to a boyfriend from a more senior class. Because they had been hitherto inseparable, Kate has not made any other close friends and now found it quite easy to isolate herself without fear of intrusion. She idealized her religious studies teacher and became very interested in world religions, strengthening her vegetarian principles.

These were some of the background events which led to the showdown with her mother, when Kate was asked to be a bridesmaid at her cousin's wedding. Kate had been wearing over-sized jumpers, short socks, long skirts and heavy shoes for some time, and mother was deeply shocked when, after much prevarication by Kate, she accompanied her to the dressmaker to be measured for her bridesmaid's dress, and saw for the first time how thin she was. Kate's mother recollected how she would spend hours bargaining in the evenings with Kate about the foods she would eat, driving miles at weekends to specialist food shops to buy the correct brands of rice, beans and spices, while Kate continued to lose weight.

Kate's mother gradually recognized that she had allowed Kate to take over many of her mothering functions for the family after her husband left home, and that she had felt unable to challenge Kate or exert the authority which her husband had always done. Kate had been a 'very good girl' during her mother's post-natal depression. She had learned to bathe her sister and change her nappies and clothes. The family therapist supported Kate's mother in asserting her responsibility and restoring balance in the family. It was impossible to engage her father in family work after the second session, but he subsequently agreed to pay Kate's fees for therapy. A good deal of grief and anger were expressed by Kate's mother and her daughters about father's departure, and there was discussion of the problems of allowing men into their home, whether they might be the mother's or her daughter's friends.

8 June – 12 July

Kate achieved her expected weight gain and her target weight (Figure 11.4). Her consultant referred her to a psychotherapist and Kate planned to return to school in September. She was due to be discharged from hospital three days after her birthday on 14 July. Among the reasons for recommending that Kate had individual psychotherapy was the belief that her mother also needed individual therapy and attention for herself, freeing her to meet her own needs.

Kate's nurses had been very impressed by her growing willingness to explore difficult areas of her life, but one of the most enjoyable aspects of her recovery was that they were able to go out with her and carry out ordinary activities, ranging from roller-skating to going to the cinema. In doing so, they were able to deal with Kate's wish to make friends with them as opposed to maintaining a professional relationship. They felt that her determination and honesty would help her to keep her appointments and to do the travelling necessary to see her therapist three times a week.

Kate was eventually discharged home. She returned to school and attended her therapy for a further 3 years, stopping when she started at university. She was followed up by the ward team and had a key worker who had been her primary nurse. Kate would drop in at weekends to see her nurse, mostly for additional support when things became difficult at home or her therapist went on holiday. Her weight has remained stable, though about 3 kg below the average.

Summary

The nursing care of Kate attempted to provide for her a setting firstly where she was safe and where her physical well-being was paramount, and secondly, where she could begin to recognize and understand some of the events in her life which had driven her to seek the solution that she experienced in anorexia nervosa. The multidisciplinary clinical team attempted to provide multidimensional interventions and interactions which were varied enough to do justice to the complexity of Kate's predicament, but which were integrated enough (through the framework of the levels of psychotherapy) to give Kate an idea of what 'good enough' parenting was like. Having this experience eventually enabled her to renegotiate with her mother her place in the reconstructed family and to begin her adolescent development assisted by a therapist, and assured that her mother was receiving the help she needed. Her elder sister received counselling for a number of years. Her younger sister adjusted well to adolescence and has done well at school.

References

American Psychiatric Association (1987). *Diagnostic and Statistical Manual of Mental Disorders*, 3rd edition, revised, DSM– 111–R. American Psychiatric Association, Washington DC.

Atkinson RL, Atkinson RC, Smith EE, *et al.* (1987). *Introduction to Psychology*, 9th edition. Harcourt Brace Jovanovich, San Diego.

Ayllon T and Haughton E (1964). Modification of symptomatic verbal behaviour of mental patients. *Behaviour Research and Therapy*; 2: 87–97.

Barnes GG (1984). *Working with Families*. Macmillan, London.

Bassøe HH and Esklund (1982). A prospective study of 133 patients with anorexia nervosa: treatment and outcome. *Acta Psychiatrica Scandinavica*; 65(2): 127–33.

Bion WR (1970). *Attention and Interpretation*. Tavistock, London.

Bossert S, Schnabel E, Krieg J-C *et al.* (1988). Modifications and problems of behavioural inpatient management of anorexia nervosa: a 'patient-suited' approach. *Acta Psychiatrica Scandinavica*; 77: 105–10.

Bowlby J (1973). *Attachment and Loss Volume 2: Separation: Anxiety and Anger*. Hogarth, London.

Bowlby J (1979). *The Making and Breaking of Affectional Bonds*. Tavistock, London.

Bowlby J (1980). *Attachment and Loss Volume 3: Loss*. Hogarth Press, London.

Boyle MP, Koff E and Gudas LJ (1981). Assessment and management of anorexia nervosa. *American Journal of Maternal Child Nursing*; 6(6): 412–8.

Bruch H (1978). *The Golden Cage*. Harvard University Press, Cambridge, Mass., USA.

Bruch H (1981). Developmental considerations of anorexia nervosa and obesity. *Canadian Journal of Psychiatry*; 26(4): 212–7.

Bruch H (1982). Anorexia nervosa: therapy and theory. *American Journal of Psychiatry*; 139(12): 1531–8.

Bryant SO and Kopeski LM (1986). Psychiatric nursing assessment of the eating disorder client. *Topics in Clinical Nursing*; 8(1): 57–66.

Carino CM and Chmelko P (1983). Disorders of eating in adolescents: anorexia nervosa and bulimia. *Nursing Clinics of North America*; 18(2): 343–52.

Cawley RH (1976). *Assumptions and preconceptions about psychotherapy*. Paper delivered to the Association of University Teachers of Psychiatry, Conference on the Teaching of Psychotherapy.

Chambers K and Yong C (1985). Management of the child with severe anorexia nervosa: multi-disciplinary approach. *Nursing*; 2(40): 1189–1200.

Clark WG (1983). Anorexia nervosa. *New Zealand Nurses Journal*; 76(2): 4–6.

Crisp AH (1980). *Anorexia Nervosa: Let Me Be*. Academic Press, London.

Crisp AH (1984). Therapeutic outcome in anorexia nervosa. *Canadian Journal of Psychiatry*; 26(4): 232–5.

Dec GW, Biederman J and Hougen TJ (1987). Cardiovascular findings in adolescent inpatients with anorexia nervosa. *Psychosomatic Medicine*; 49(3): 285–90.

Diem K and Lentner C (1970). *Scientific Tables*. Geigy (UK) Ltd, Macclesfield.

Feighner JP, Robins E, Guze SB *et al.* (1972). Criteria for use in psychiatric research. *Archives of General Psychiatry*; 26: 57–63.

Frisch RE and McArthur JW (1974). Menstrual cycles: fatness as a determinant of minimum weight for height necessary for their maintenance or onset. *Science*; 13 Sep 74: 949–51.

Garner DM (1981). Body image in anorexia nervosa. *Canadian Journal of Psychiatry*; 26(4): 224–31.

Garner DM and Garfinkel PE (1979). The Eating Attitudes Test: an index of the symptoms of anorexia nervosa. *Psychological Medicine*; 9: 273–9.

Garner DM and Garfinkel PE (1980). Socio-cultural factors in the development of anorexia nervosa. *Psychological Medicine*; 10: 647–56.

Garner DM, Garfinkel PE and Bonato DP (1987). Body image measurement in eating disorders. *Advances in Psychosomatic Medicine*; 17: 119–33.

Garner DM, Olmstead MP, Bohr V *et al.* (1982) The Eating Attitudes Test: psychometric features and clinical correlates. *Psychological Medicine*; 12: 871–8.

Goodsitt A (1985). Self-psychology and the treatment of anorexia nervosa; in Garner DM and Garfinkel PE (eds) *Handbook of Psychotherapy for Anorexia Nervosa and Bulimia*. Guilford Press, New York.

Gordon M (1982). *Nursing Diagnosis: Process and Application*. McGraw Hill, New York.

Gull WW (1894). *A Collection of the Published Writings of William Withey Gull*. The New Sydenham Society, London.

Harding SE (1985). Anorexia nervosa. *Pediatric Nursing*; 11(4): 275–7.

Hartman A and Laird J (1983). *Family-Centred Social Work Practice*. Free Press, New York.

Heron JM and Leheup RF (1984). Happy families? *British Journal of Psychiatry*; 145: 136–8.

Horne M and Gallen M (1987). Anorexia nervosa: an object relations approach to primary treatment. *British Journal of Psychiatry*; 151: 192–4.

Hsu LKG (1986). The treatment of anorexia nervosa. *American Journal of Psychiatry*; 143: 573–81.

Huon G and Brown LB (1984). Psychological correlates of weight control among anorexia nervosa patients and normal girls. *British Journal of Medical Psychology*; 57(1): 61–6.

Huse DM and Lucas AR (1984). Dietary patterns in anorexia nervosa. *American Journal of Clinical Nutrition*; 40(2): 251–4.

Jackson MA (1981). *Inpatient treatment of anorexia nervosa*. Unpublished paper.

Johnson-Sabine, Wood K, Patton G *et al.* (1988). Abnormal eating attitudes in London schoolgirls – a prospective epidemiological study. *Psychological Medicine*; 18: 615–22.

Kalucy RS, Crisp AH and Harding B (1977). A study of 56 families with anorexia nervosa. *British Journal of Medical Psychology*; 50: 381–95.

Keys A, Brozek J, Henesehel A *et al.* (1950). *The Biology of Human Starvation*. University of Minnesota Press, Minneapolis, USA.

King SH (1972). Coping and growth. *Seminars in Psychiatry*; 4(4): 355–66.

King MB and Bhugra D (1989). Eating disorders: lessons from a cross-cultural study. *Psychological Medicine*; 19: 955–8.

Krølner B and Toft B (1983). Vertebral bone loss: an unheeded side effect of therapeutic bed rest. *Clinical Science*; 64: 537–40.

Lewis KG (1989) The use of colour-coded genograms in family therapy. *Journal of Marital and Family Therapy*; 15(2): 169–76.

Lilly GE and Sanders JB (1987). Nursing management of anorexic adolescents. *Journal of Psychosocial Nursing and Mental Health Services*; 25(11): 30–3.

Mann AH, Wakeling A, Wood K *et al.* (1983). Screening for abnormal eating attitudes and psychiatric morbidity in an unselected population of 15-year-old schoolgirls. *Psychological Medicine*; 13: 573–80.

Margo JL (1985). Anorexia nervosa in adolescents. *British*

Journal of Medical Psychology; **58(2)**: 193–5.

Martin F (1983). Subgroups in anorexia nervosa: a family systems study, in Darby PL *et al.* (eds), *Anorexia Nervosa: Recent Developments in Research*, Alan R Liss, New York.

McNamara RJ (1982). The role of the nurse at the bedside. *Canadian Nurse*; **78(10)**: 35–40

Minuchin S (1974). *Families and Family Therapy*. Tavistock, London.

Minuchin S (1978). *Psychosomatic Families: Anorexia Nervosa in Context.* Harvard University Press, Cambridge, Mass., USA.

Misik IM (1981). When the anorexic patient challenges you. *Nursing*; **11(12)**: 46–9.

Morgan HG, Purgold J, Welbourne J (1983). Management and outcome in anorexia nervosa: a standardised prognostic study. *British Journal of Psychiatry*; **43**: 282–7.

Morgan HG and Russell GFM (1975). Value of family background and clinical features as predictors of long-term outcome in anorexia nervosa: four-year follow-up study of 41 patients. *Psychological Medicine*; **5**: 355–71.

Orbach S (1978). *Fat is a Feminist Issue.* Paddington Press, New York.

Orbach S (1985). Accepting the symptoms: a feminist psycho-analytic treatment of anorexia nervosa, in Garner DM and Garfinkel PE (eds), *Handbook of Psychotherapy for Anorexia Nervosa and Bulimia.* Guilford Press, New York.

Orr R (1979). Anorexia nervosa: a self-imposed starvation. *Nursing Care*; **9(10)**: 28–31.

Palmer RL (1980). *Anorexia Nervosa.* Penguin, Harmondsworth, Middlesex.

Piazza E, Piazza N and Rollins N (1980). Anorexia nervosa: controversial aspects of therapy. *Comprehensive Psychiatry*; **21(3)**: 177–89.

Raymond CA (1987). Long-term sequelae pondered in anorexia nervosa. *Journal of the American Medical Association*; **257(24)**: 3324–5.

Rieger W, Brady JP and Weiberg E (1978). Haematologic changes in anorexia nervosa. *American Journal of Psychiatry*; **135(8)**: 984–5.

Ritter S (1988). Care plan for an anxious person, based on Cawley's levels of psychotherapy, in Collister B (ed) *Person to Person.* Edward Arnold, London.

Ritter S (1989). *The Bethlem Royal and Maudsley Hospital Manual of Clinical Psychiatric Nursing Principles and Procedures.* Harper and Row, London.

Rollins N and Blackwell A (1968). The treatment of anorexia nervosa in children and adolescents: stage 1. *Journal of Child Psychology and Psychiatry*; **9**: 81–91.

Roberts A, Mandin H and Roxburgh P (1986). Unexplained seizure in anorexia nervosa. *Canadian Journal of Psychiatry*; **31**: 653–5.

Rubin RL (1986). Assisting adolescents toward mental health. *Nursing Clinics of North America*; **21(3)**: 439–50.

Russell GFM (1977). General management of anorexia nervosa and difficulties in assessing the efficacy of treatment, in Vigersky R (ed) *Anorexia Nervosa.* Raven Press, New York.

Russell GFM (1983). Anorexia nervosa and bulimia nervosa, in Russell GFM and Hersov LA (eds), *Handbook of Psychiatry*, Cambridge University Press.

Russell GFM and Mezey AG (1962). An analysis of weight gain in patients with anorexia nervosa treated with high-calorie diets. *Clinical Science*; **23**: 449–61.

Russell GFM, Szmukler GI, Dare C and Eisler I (1987). An evaluation of family therapy in anorexia nervosa and bulimia. *Archives of General Psychiatry*; **44(12)**: 1047–56.

Rycroft C (1968). *A Critical Dictionary of Psychoanalysis.* Penguin, Harmondsworth, Middlesex.

Sansone RA, Fine MA and Chew R (1988). A longitudinal analysis of the experiences of nursing staff on an inpatient eating disorders unit. *International Journal of Eating Disorders*; **7(1)**: 124–31.

Schleimer K (1983). Dieting in teenage schoolgirls: a longitudinal prospective study. *Acta Paediatrica Scandinavica*; **312**: 1–54.

Schlemmer JK and Barnett PA (1977). Management of manipulative behaviour of anorexia nervosa patients. *Journal of Psychiatric Nursing and Mental Health Services*; **15(11)**: 35–7.

Schwartz DM, Thompson MG and Johnson CL (1982). Anorexia nervosa and bulimia: the sociocultural context. *International Journal of Eating Disorders*. **1(3)**: 20–36.

Silverman JA (1989). Louis-Victor Marcé, 1828–1864: anorexia nervosa's forgotten man. *Psychological Medicine*; **19**: 835–933.

Skinner BF (1957). *Verbal Behaviour.* Appleton-Century Croft, New York.

Sloan G and Leichner P (1986). Is there a relationship between sexual abuse or incest and eating disorders? *Canadian Journal of Psychiatry*; **31**: 656–60.

Snow JT and Harris MB (1989). Disordered eating in South-Western Pueblo Indians and Hispanics. *Journal of Adolescence*; **12**: 329–36.

Steinhausen H-C and Glanville K (1983). Follow-up studies of anorexia nervosa: a review of research findings. *Psychological Medicine*; **13**: 239–49.

Szmukler GI, Berkowitz R, Eisler I *et al.* (1987). Expressed emotion in individual and family settings: a comparative study. *British Journal of Psychiatry*; **151**: 174–8.

Theander S (1983). Research on outcome and prognosis of anorexia nervosa and some results from a Swedish long-term study. *International Journal of Eating Disorders*; **2(4)**: 167–74.

Tolstrup K, Brinch M, Isoger T *et al.* (1985). Long-term outcome of 151 cases of anorexia nervosa. *Acta Psychiatrica Scandinavica*; **71(4)**: 380–7.

Touyz SW, Beumont JV, Collins JK *et al.* (1984). Body shape perception and its disturbance in anorexia nervosa. *British Journal of Psychiatry*; **144**: 167–71.

Vandereycken W (1985). In-patient treatment of anorexia nervosa: some research-guided changes. *Journal of Psychiatric Research*; **19(2/3)**: 413–22.

Williams M (1982). Anorexia nervosa – milieu therapy of young adolescents. *Australian Nurses Journal*; **11(8)**: 38–40.

Williams P (1986). Unpublished upgrading paper.

Winnicott DW (1965). *Maturational Processes and the Facilitating Environment.* International Psychoanalytic Library, London.

Wooley DW and Wooley S (1982). The Beverly Hills eating disorder: the mass marketing of anorexia nervosa. *International Journal of Eating Disorders*; **1(3)**: 57–69.

Wright SJ (1986). Altered body image in anorexia nervosa. *Professional Nurse*; **1(1)**: 260–2.

Yager J (1982). Family issues in the pathogenesis of anorexia nervosa. *Psycosomatic Medicine*; **44(1)**: 43–60.

Further reading

Bowlby J (1969). *Attachment and Loss Volume 1: Attachment.* Hogarth, London.

Casper RC and Davis JM (1977). On the course of anorexia nervosa. *American Journal of Psychiatry*; 134: 974–8.

Gillies C and Russell GFM (1983). Nursing treatment, in Russell GFM and Hersov LA (eds), *Handbook of Psychiatry*. Cambridge University Press.

Hsu LKG (1983). The etiology of anorexia nervosa. *Psychological Medicine*; 13: 231–8.

Offer D, Ostrov E and Howard KI (1981). The mental health professional's concept of the normal adolescent. *Archives of General Psychiatry*; 38: 149–52.

Peplau H (1952). *Interpersonal Relations in Nursing*. GP Putnams and Sons, New York.

Pierloot R, Vandereyken W and Verhaest S (1982). An inpatient treatment programme for anorexia nervosa patients. *Acta Psychiatrica Scandinavica*; 66: 1–8.

Toner BB, Garfinkel PE and Garner DE (1986). Long-term follow-up of anorexia nervosa. *Psychosomatic Medicine*; 48(7): 520–9.

Wardle J (1986). Eating style: a validation study of the Dutch eating behaviour questionnaire in normal subjects and women with eating disorders. *Journal of Psychosomatic Research*; 31(2): 61–9.

12

Caring for a child with chronic illness using King's theory of nursing
Dorothy Whyte

Imogene King is one of the early American nursing theorists; her first book *Toward a Theory for Nursing* was published in 1971 and updated in 1981. The development of her theory in the context of family nursing is discussed and illustrated in a review of theoretical approaches to family health (Clements and Roberts, 1983). In this chapter I shall briefly discuss chronic illness, outline the major concepts and assumptions of King's theory, and then demonstrate its application to the assessment and care of Stephen who is 11 years old and has cystic fibrosis.

Chronic illness

The word 'chronic' encompasses the concept of time, and the Shorter Oxford Dictionary defines it as lingering or lasting a long time. Mattson's (1972) definition is also helpful:

'Chronic illness refers to a disorder with a protracted course which can be progressive and fatal or associated with a relatively normal life span despite impaired physical and mental functioning. Such a disease frequently shows periods of acute exacerbations requiring intensive medical attention.'

(p.801)

Cystic fibrosis (CF) is a permanent non-curable inherited condition. It is estimated that around 400 new CF cases are diagnosed each year in the United Kingdom, and in 1984 there were an estimated 6,000 sufferers (Capewell, 1986). The defective gene has just been located, after many years of intensive research (Editorial, 1989). While the discovery will have early application in terms of accurate diagnosis and screening, Lap-Chee Tsui, one of the scientists who achieved the breakthrough, acknowledges that it will require a long period of research and development before therapy aimed at the specific defect becomes available. It is likely therefore that care of children and young people with the disease and their families will remain an important nursing commitment for many years to come.

The principal effects of the disease are seen in the lungs and respiratory tract, the digestive system and the sweat. It is the susceptibility to respiratory infections which becomes debilitating and life-threatening. The vigorous physiotherapy, supervision of diet and medication replacing the digestive enzymes place a considerable burden upon a family's coping mechanisms. It is the grim prognosis, however, which impinges most painfully upon the family experience. Even with early diagnosis and vigorous treatment, most patients with CF die before their thirtieth birthday and some still die in early childhood. The essential characteristics then are of a pathological condition which can be treated but not cured, which is long-term but with a varying course, which requires intensive daily therapy in order to maintain a reasonable quality as well as quantity of life – and which is ultimately for the study of chronic illness in childhood, its impact upon families and the nature of nursing support.

King's theory of nursing

King's theory suggests that:

'It is humanistic, realistic, and basic to understanding behaviours in human interaction which is the foundation of nursing practice.'
(Clements and Roberts, 1983, p.177)

It was the focus on interaction which drew me to it, at a point in my work with a family where I had used an activities of living model (Roper *et al.*, 1985) for assessment, but found that once I wanted to go beyond physical symptoms and practical problems to the more complex area of interacting with families in a supportive relationnnship, the activities of living approach was inadequate.

I liked King's definition of health:

'Health is defined as dynamic life experiences of a human being, which implies continuous adjustment to stressors in the internal and external environment through optimum use of one's resources to achieve maximum potential for daily living. Health relates to the way individuals deal with the stresses of growth and development while functioning within the cultural pattern in which they were born and to which they attempt to conform.'
(King, 1981 p.4–5)

King contends that the goal of nursing is 'concern for the health of individuals and the health care of groups'. A major assumption of her work is that nurses and patients generally communicate information, mutually set goals, and take action to attain goals. She utilizes systems theory with the premise that 'human beings are open systems interacting with the environment' (p.10) as a basis for her conceptual framework for nursing.

Systems theory

While general systems theory as proposed by von Bertalanffy (1968) has not attained the status of a complete theory of knowledge, it has influenced the development of theoretical frameworks in a range of disciplines from business studies and information technology to sociology and nursing. Skynner (1976) suggests that it represents a new conceptual leap in scientific development, providing a new way of viewing phenomena in their total relationships rather than in isolation from one another. A brief review of the major concepts of systems thinking indicates their relevance to nursing work with families.

The concept of wholeness is important, not just holistic care of the child who has the illness, but a holistic view of the family and the relationship of its parts. The boundaries which separate the sub-systems – child from siblings, child from parents, parents from each other – affect family interaction and are important too in separating the family system from the social system of which it remains a part. The permeability of the boundary may have profound implications for the health of family functioning. Over time it will become apparent how the family maintains homeostasis, a steady state achieved in spite of environmental stresses. Negative feedback helps to maintain stability by balancing the input and output of the system (Clements and Roberts, 1983). For example, when a spell of illness has the effect of causing a husband to give extra attention to the sick child and to share the burden of care with his wife, this has the negative feedback effect of damping down the stress levels to more manageable proportions. The reverse happens when the husband opts out leaving his wife to cope unsupported with the increased demand for care, thus providing positive feedback and pushing the system further away from stability.

The nurse is herself (or himself) a sub-system within the health care system. In her contact with families she may at times be drawn in or choose to enter the family system, affecting its homeostasis or stability. She could provide a negative feedback effect in the situation illustrated above, by compensating to some extent for the husband's defection in providing emotional and practical support to the overburdened mother. More effectively, she may be able to help the husband to confront the reasons for his own behaviour and to find a more adaptive response which will contribute to family stability.

King's theory is based upon a consideration of dynamically interacting systems which she termed personal, interpersonal and social systems. These she linked with major concepts:

- Personal systems: Individuals, interacting with the environment; understood by examining concepts of perception, self, body image, growth and development, time and space.
- Interpersonal systems: two or more individuals interacting; understood by examining such concepts as role, interaction, communication, transaction and stress.
- Social systems: dynamic forces within society that influence health and behaviour; understood by examining such concepts as organization, power, authority, status, decision making and role. (pp. 10–12).

The concepts are inter-related and influence every person's behaviour. Used as a guide to assessment they can provide a valuable data base on the patient or family, can assist in the identification of problems and help in the setting of goals to resolve problems.

Case study

For the purpose of writing this chapter, I have isolated a time segment from a six year involvement with this family. The first child in the family died at the age of seventeen months due to CF. The parents, Donald and Mary, worked painfully through to a resolution of their grief and two years later Lesley was born. She was healthy and gave great joy. Their son Stephen was born two years later and a diagnosis of CF was confirmed when he was nine months old.

The segment relates to a particular crisis point in the family's experience at a time when Stephen was eleven years of age and Lesley was thirteen. It was precipitated by an intercurrent infection requiring hospital admission. Illness invariably affected

Stephen's mood and behaviour and his irritability with his mother reduced her to tears. The ward sister felt that marital tension was worsening the situation and voiced her concern to me. My offer to visit the home that evening was accepted by Mary. The data which I had already gathered on the family provide essential background information.

An assessment of Stephen's problems was undertaken using an activities of living framework (Roper *et al.*, 1985).

Eating and drinking: Stephen became anorexic whenever he was unwell; at these times trying to persuade him to finish his meals was a source of tension.

Eliminating: his stools were mostly normal, 2 times per day; sometimes they were 'porridgy' looking and occasionally he would have 4–5 stools per day. When they were loose at these times they were smelly, and Stephen found this embarrassing at school.

Breathing: Stephen coughed a lot and expectorated. This caused some friction at school, where one class-mate said, 'Watch, you'll poison the ground'. He was very interested in physiotherapy and listened to the explanations he was given. He had taught a neighbour how to perform it and also his aunt, when he stayed with her overnight.

Mobility: He enjoyed football and other sports but tired fairly quickly, particularly at the times when he was less well. He tended to try to prove himself in this area and a recent school report said, 'Stephen takes a very active part in physical education classes'. His mother worried about him getting wet; she discouraged swimming and usually drove him to school by car, although it was within fairly easy walking distance.

Personal hygiene: Stephen was well able to manage his own personal hygiene but his mother tended to help him because he took so long about it.

Working and playing: Stephen was an intelligent boy who did not at that stage enjoy school but nevertheless coped fairly easily with it.

Maintaining a safe environment: there were the normal hazards of childhood and the need for safety in the home, on the roads and at school. In addition, to maintain optimum health in the face of chronic illness it was important that he should have physiotherapy at least three times per day, antibiotic and enzyme treatment and a nutritious diet.

Communicating: Stephen had a quick tongue and a lively sense of humour. He could be very irritable at times with his family, particularly with his mother, but was also very affectionate. He became a firm favourite with hospital staff who enjoyed his fun and teasing, although one or two members of staff found his cheekiness difficult to manage.

Sleeping was not usually a problem, although when he was less well coughing could be disturbing to him and his parents.

Expressing sexuality: Stephen was already interested in his appearance and had a 'girl-friend' in his class.

Dying: the life-threatening nature of his illness was not kept from him and his parents encouraged his questions, but he usually preferred not to speak about it. His awareness of the prognosis was indicated in give-away remarks such as one made to the play leader at a time when he was anxious to get home in time for his birthday. When she said that it could be worse, he could have a party in the ward, he said, 'What could be worse, tell me, what could be worse?' When she did not answer he said, 'You could be dead for your birthday. I wish my Mum would come. Do you think I could 'phone her?'

King's framework extends the assessment.

Personal system

Self: As an individual, Stephen was a fighter who made light of his limitations and maintained an optimistic approach to life except on the few occasions when he reached a very low ebb. He was interested in his treatment and most of the time he complied with the demanding regime.

Body image: He took an intelligent interest in his body, thought out explanations for changes, and had his own ideas about treatment decisions. Soon after he changed to Creon as his replacement enzyme treatment he said delightedly to his mother, 'Now my jobbies are like everyone else's'. He did not like being small for his age and weighed himself every day. During a good spell when he was gaining weight he said, 'Maybe I'll soon be able to wear size

9–10 clothes. I wouldn't care what I had if I was just a bit bigger and a bit fatter'.

Perception: When he won first prize for disco dancing he began planning a career in show business. His mother was a bit dubious and suggested that the smokey atmosphere might not agree with him. He dismissed that airily with the pronouncement, 'I'll have the cure by then'. He was aware, however, of how hard he had to fight to keep on top. At one stage he had fallen from the top of his class to the bottom due to time in hospital, and was assessed by the educational psychologist. The outcome was that he seemed to be keeping up at present but if necessary he could be offered remedial classes in the future. His reaction was, 'I'm not having remedial, I'd just give up'.

Stephen's perception of himself was closely linked with his *body image* and his personal construction of his illness as something to be overcome. Growth has been seen to be something of a preoccupation, as CF children are typically small in stature and slow in sexual development. Their physical abilities, however, are limited only by their respiratory problems. Emotional development was inevitably influenced to some extent by the parental anxiety surrounding him, but he had considerable self-confidence and related well to his peers. Intellectual development was hampered only by the interruption to schooling caused by illness.

Time was a very important concept in Stephen's life. Time in hospital was time lost from other things. Most of his hospital stays were shadowed by events he might miss if he did not get out in time – an important football match, a concert, a birthday. As he began to enjoy school more and to work hard, he began to worry about losing time at school which might lead to his losing the ground he had gained. As mentioned already, the possibility of time running out for him, or of his situation being changed by the discovery of a cure were present in his awareness.

The concept of *space* in relation to the welfare of a child relates to freedom to explore the environment, to engage in physical exercise and to preserve some personal space within the environment. This involves moving from the dependence of early childhood to the independence of adulthood. Chronic illness can impose severe limitations on this normal development, but in Stephen's case there was a conscious effort on the part of his parents to allow him to achieve greater independence. At eleven he was the youngest child to go on the CF adventure camp. The fact that trained staff were in attendance provided a sense of security for this venture. He was encouraged to take physical exercise and had recently been learning to play badminton with his father. He had his own room at home and in hospital his need for personal space was respected. He was always cared for in one of two side-rooms where he could entertain his visitors with a degree of privacy.

Interpersonal system

Stephen was secure in his *role* as the younger child and the only son in the family. He was quicker than his older sister who often resented the attention that her brother's illness demanded. These demands affected *family interaction* and created considerable *stress*. His mother said on more than one occasion, 'The only rows in this house are about Stephen and his physio'. Stephen's father took over the evening physiotherapy after a particularly stressful time when Mary felt that she was having to cope with everything and it was too much. The difficulties were not removed by this *transaction* because Stephen often reported to his mother that Donald had not been doing it properly. 'He's looking out the window and not looking at what he's doing.' This upset Mary who would then let fly at Donald with a comment like, 'It's his life that's at stake – it's up to you'. Having sparked off the row, Stephen would sit back and watch television while his parents fought over him.

While both parents were strongly motivated towards family life there were times when the demanding situation produced role strain, particularly for Donald, who found it quite difficult to deal with the discontinuity of his everyday working life and the intense demands of life at home, which he felt were quite incomprehensible to his workmates. *Communication* between Stephen and his parents, particularly his mother, was open and she encouraged him to share his fears if she sensed that something was worrying him. Indeed, the dyadic

relationship between mother and son was possibly too close, due to the demands of treatment and of periods of illness, but the *disequilibrium* which this could cause in the family system was offset by the quality of the spouse sub-system. Mary and Donald had developed considerable strengths through the death of their eldest child early in their marriage and although Mary sometimes wished they could share their feelings more, they usually managed to overcome any major blocks in communication and to move forward together again. The greatest communication difficulty was probably with the healthy sibling, Lesley. As suggested by Burton (1975) parental preoccupation with Stephen was interpreted by her as rejection, and through the years she often made comments like, 'If he asked for it, he'd get it'. Lesley was quiet and possibly had a diminished sense of self-worth due to the attention given to Stephen and the fact that he was obviously more intelligent than she was. She seldom asked questions or expressed feelings about Stephen's illness.

Social system

The social system for this family consisted of an informal support network provided in part by extended family, but more by friends in the neighbourhood and a church group who provided practical help at times in the form of baby-sitting and spiritual support through prayer. Within the social system were groups like Boys' Brigade and a football club. The family boundary was sufficiently permeable to allow some sharing of the burden, but sufficiently closed to maintain the integrity of the family unit. The Cystic Fibrosis Research Trust[*] provided information and Donald was actively involved in its fund-raising activities, but Mary found the contact with other sufferers of CF too threatening because of the tendency to compare their progress or deterioration with Stephen's condition. The formal support network included the health care team, in the form of hospital staff and myself as home visiting nurse; the general prac-

[*] Cystic Fibrosis Research Trust, Alexandria House, 5 Blyth Road, Bromley, Kent BR1 3RS. Tel: (081) 464 7211.

titioner was consulted on general health matters but the hospital team were seen as the experts in management of CF.

The complex interplay of the concepts of *power* and *authority* with *status* and *decision-making* were illustrated by the way in which Stephen's health needs were dealt with by the school system. At one stage Mary was concerned that Stephen was not adequately managing his own physiotherapy (by the forced expiratory technique) and requested supervision. In most instances there is a member of school staff able to take on such a task, but in Stephen's school, the headmaster explained the difficulties experienced with lunch-time supervision of the pupils, and stated that there was no-one to whom he could delegate the responsibility. In my role as home visiting nurse, I made contact with the community nursing supervisor, the community physiotherapist, the community paediatrician, the school nursing supervisor and the health visiting service. It seemed that, while there was sympathy for the situation, no-one was able to take on the daily commitment of supervision. A meeting was called by the school doctor which included the community physiotherapist, the school nurse, the headmaster, Mary and myself. The difficulty was discussed and I had to resist, on Mary's behalf, the suggestion that she should come up to the school every lunch-time to supervise Stephen. The physiotherapist offered to come whenever Stephen's condition had worsened, indicating a need for chest percussion, but her workload did not allow her to visit daily. Power in this situation was unmistakeably in the hands of the headmaster who seemed to have total authority within his domain. It struck me that an irrational but real factor in his decision-making was revulsion for sputum. On more than one occasion he said, 'I mean, it's not a very nice thing to ask anyone to do'.

In the end a rather make-shift arrangement was cobbled together, whereby I went in one day per week, and the school nurse covered another day. A record was kept of the length of time the session took Stephen, and the nature of the sputum. At first covertly, but later with the headmaster's permission, the school janitor, who had an excellent relationship with Stephen and with the other children, looked in to see how Stephen was managing on the other days. It is, however, a matter of some concern that, while the principle of educating children with special needs alongside healthy children has been officially adopted, the school and health care systems are not always able or willing to respond to a need for special care in school.

Family crisis

Golan (1969) described crisis as having four elements: the hazardous event, the vulnerable state, the precipitating factor and the state of active crisis. In the presence of a hazardous event such as the presence of life-threatening illness in a child, a family becomes vulnerable. It then may require quite a minor precipitating factor to throw the family into disequilibrium. As one mother put it, 'You're walking a tightrope of coping all the time'. It was in this case quite a minor event which produced a crisis.

Mary recounted how she had gone in to the ward that day, taking Stephen's football album. She was already tired and tense, wondering how his mood would be. As soon as she sat down he started looking for his stickers.

'Where are my stickers?' he demanded.

'I don't know – think where you had them last.'

'Help me then' he shouted.

She reacted inwardly, 'No, I won't help him'. She felt deep down she wanted him to fight the illness, not to give in to it.

He said,

'Och, I'm fed up with this. I wish I wasnae here'.

She rounded on him then. 'Do you think I've worked for you all these eleven years just for you to give up?'

He took that in. The tension and the stress of confrontation took its toll, however, and soon after that Mary was in tears in the duty room.

As we discussed it at home, I identified and validated with the parents that they resist any attempt by Stephen to adopt the sick role.

I asked, 'You feel he's seeing himself as ill?'

'Yes, that's it.'

I suggested that from Stephen's point of view the way they were dealing with his behaviour was probably about right; he felt safe to let out his anger and frustration at his mother, which was preferable to his turning in on himself and becoming withdrawn and depressed. He could then relate to his father's bantering approach. Donald recalled a conversation a few days earlier at home, in which Stephen was feeling low and moaning, 'Why me?' Donald pointed out another child who was paralysed, who had been in the news recently, and said, 'You're going to get better, there are plenty worse off than you'. That tactic seemed to lift Stephen's mood, and Donald implied that Mary was too sympathetic with him, that she 'mothered' him too much, and perhaps should use what he called a 'jokey' approach. I felt that it was important to see the two approaches as complementary, as each seemed to fulfil an important function in supporting Stephen. One accepted the need to regress at times of stress, while the other encouraged a positive attitude to the situation. (See Rose, 1984 for a detailed discussion of childrens' coping strategies).

Stephen's self-perception was important, and most of the time he strove to live a normal life and refused to see himself as disabled. When he felt really ill, his perception changed and he showed a sense of defeat. If his regression took the form of cuddling in to his mother it was accepted, but if he expressed anger or hopelessness his parents refused to accept his construction of the situation. This led to conflict and stress within the family system, but can be seen as constructive in terms of adaptation to illness. It was, however, emotionally very draining and it seemed important to find ways in which Mary particularly could be helped with the burden of care. We agreed that the weep in the duty room was probably a good thing, providing a safety valve for suppressed emotion. We looked together at the regular issue of contention, the evening physiotherapy sessions. I suggested that it was important to find some way of organizing the regime which would allow each of them some personal time. There was a sense in which each parent felt trapped by the intense demands of the situation and the lack of time for anything other than caring for Stephen. This led to fatigue and impaired communication. Donald felt too that Mary was allowing Stephen to be too dependent for

his personal care; 'He can dress himself, he does on a Saturday'. Mary admitted that she just could not stand the time it took Stephen, because he dawdled and day-dreamed, 'and it's enough of a hassle getting everything done in the morning'. She agreed, however, that it would pay off in the long run if she could just expect him to get dressed himself, i.e. leave him to it without nagging.

Since Stephen's well-being so profoundly affected the whole family, we also discussed ways in which he could be helped to cope with the frustrations of weakness and of being in hospital. Mary suggested that if he could be asked to undertake some art project for the ward it would present him with a challenge and keep him occupied. There was some concern also about Lesley, who had been very weepy in recent days. While Stephen was in hospital she frequently went to a friend's house after school and stayed there for tea. We discussed the need to ensure that she had some time each week when each parent gave her individual attention.

The nursing intervention can be summarized by using King's goal-oriented nursing record. This requires identification of a problem and the setting of a goal as a transaction between nurse and client. Since assessment necessarily precedes this step, and since evaluation of the extent to which the goal has been attained is essential in follow-up, the theory clearly incorporates the nursing process.

Critique of the model

King views the maintenance of health as a continuous adaptation to stress and contends that the 'family, as a social system, and health, as a goal for nursing, are two major concepts in the framework and in the theory of nursing' (in Clements, 1983, p. 178). This model, therefore, unambiguously sets health care support in the context of a partnership with families and, therefore, has the potential for application with families caring for a chronically sick member. Indeed, I felt that King's theory helped me to make a full assessment of the family situation and to make a more purposeful contribution to care. In a long-term supportive nursing relationship with a family it would not seem

	Goal	Plan	Evaluation
Problem I (Objective) Stephen's dependence. (Subjective) 'It's such a hassle in the morning'.	Stephen will dress himself daily.	Mother will make clear that the task is Stephen's.	Check at next visit if goal has been met.
Problem II (Objective) Parents' stress and exhaustion. (Subjective) 'I just cannae handle it'.	Allow each parent some personal time. Encourage sharing of the burden.	Stephen and Mary to agree that she should reduce her hospital visiting time. Each parent to have one free evening per week, and one evening out together per month. Physiotherapy to be shared equally, and involvement of extended family to be encouraged.	Monitor how much personal time parents manage to have.
Problem III (Objective) Lesley's sense of rejection. (Subjective) 'If he asked for it he'd get it.'	Lesley 's self-confidence will improve through increased emotional security.	One parent to have evening meal with Lesley on alternate nights while Stephen is in hospital. Time to be set aside twice a week when one parent takes Lesley out or plans a shared activity with her.	Check with parents how they feel they are meeting this goals; chat with Lesley to assess her feelings.

Figure 12.1 Care plan for Stephen and his family.

appropriate to be constantly setting goals, but a time of disequilibrium can afford an opportunity to review the effects of long-term stress, to identify specific problems and to seek to initiate change. There is evidence that people are more receptive to intervention during a period of crisis than at other times (Golan, 1969). The opportunity to talk through difficulties with an empathetic listener at such a time can facilitate communication between partners, freeing them to move forward together with new perceptions and strategies for coping with their intensely demanding situation.

A nurse in this situation is providing negative feedback, helping to reduce stress and re-establish homeostasis or stability. In chronic childhood illness the family becomes the focus of care, and relationships are a primary consideration since these are the relationships which sustain the child. A nursing model based on interaction and systems thinking is a useful tool for planning intervention.

However, King's theory has a number of shortcomings which should be acknowledged. Firstly, the theory presents nine major concepts (interaction, perception, communication, transaction, role, stress, growth and development, time and space) which makes the theory rather complex, although she defines the concepts to show interrelationships. The conceptual framework only guides the practitioner regarding an approach to care and lacks detail regarding physical care. As in this example, a comprehensive care plan for Stephen required an assessment using Roper's (1985) activities of daily living framework.

Secondly, King's theory is dependent upon patients and their families being able to interact competently with the nurse. This would exclude unconscious or confused patients and infants. It not only requires interactional skills on the part of the patient, but also considerable skills on the part of the nurse, so that moments of nurse-patient interaction realize their full potential.

Thirdly, Ackermann *et al.* (1989) state that 'because King's theory is relatively new, empirical testing is at the beginning, and it remains to be seen if relationships exist between concepts' (p.355).

However, it is clear that King's theory makes a useful contribution to nursing practice with its focus upon mutual co-operation between the patient and family and the nurse.

References

Ackermann ML, Brink SA, Clanton JA *et al.* (1989). Imogen King: theory of goal attainment, in Marriner-Tomey A (ed), *Nursing Theorists and their Work*. 2nd edn. CV Mosby, St Louis.

Burton L (1975). *The Family Life of Sick Children*. Routledge and Kegan Paul, London.

Capewell G (1986). *Cystic Fibrosis*. Office of Health Economics, London.

Clements IW and **Roberts FB** (1983). *Family Health: A Theoretical Approach to Nursing Care*. John Wiley, Chichester.

Editorial (1989). The cystic fibrosis gene is found. *Science*; **235**: 923.

Golan N (1969). When is a client in crisis? *Social Casework*; **July**: 389–94.

King I (1971). *Toward a Theory for Nursing: General Concepts of Human Behaviour*. John Wiley, Chichester.

King I (1981). *A Theory for Nursing: Systems, Concepts, Process*. John Wiley, Chichester.

Mattson A (1972). Long-term physical illness and psychological adaptation. *Pediatrics*; **50**: 801–11.

Roper N, Logan W and **Tierney A** (1985). *The Elements of Nursing*. Churchill Livingstone, Edinburgh.

Rose MH (1984). The concepts of coping and vulnerability as applied to children with chronic conditions. *Issues in Comprehensive Pediatric Nursing*; **7**: 177–86.

Skynner R (1976). *One Flesh: Separate Persons. Principles of Family and Marital Psychotherapy*. Constable, London.

Von Bertalanfy L (1968). *General Systems Theory*. Brazillier, New York.

Index